Practical Plans for Difficult Conversations in Medicine

Practical Plans for Difficult Conversations in Medicine

Strategies That Work in Breaking Bad News

ROBERT BUCKMAN, M.D., PH.D.
Medical Oncologist, Princess Margaret Hospital
Professor, University of Toronto
Toronto, Ontario, Canada
Adjunct Professor, M.D. Anderson Cancer Center,
    University of Texas
Houston, Texas

The Johns Hopkins University Press
Baltimore

The Johns Hopkins University Press
2715 North Charles Street
Baltimore, Maryland 21218-4363
www.press.jhu.edu

Library of Congress Cataloging-in-Publication Data

Buckman, Rob.
    Practical plans for difficult conversations in medicine : strategies that work in breaking bad
news / Robert Buckman.
        p. ; cm.
    Includes bibliographical references and index.
    ISBN-13: 978-0-8018-9557-9 (hardcover : alk. paper)
    ISBN-10: 0-8018-9557-X (hardcover : alk. paper)
    ISBN-13: 978-0-8018-9558-6 (pbk. : alk. paper)
    ISBN-10: 0-8018-9558-8 (pbk. : alk. paper)
    1. Physician and patient. 2. Bad news. 3. Interpersonal communication. I. Title.
    [DNLM: 1. Physician-Patient Relations. 2. Communication. 3. Physician's Role—
psychology. 4. Truth Disclosure. W 62 B925p 2010]
    R727.3.B835   2010
    610.69'6—dc22   2009038868

A catalog record for this book is available from the British Library.

*Special discounts are available for bulk purchases of this book. For more information, please
contact Special Sales at 410-516-6936 or specialsales@press.jhu.edu.*

The Johns Hopkins University Press uses environmentally friendly book materials, including
recycled text paper that is composed of at least 30 percent post-consumer waste, whenever
possible. All of our book papers are acid-free, and our jackets and covers are printed on paper
with recycled content.

To the Princess Margaret Hospital and the University of Toronto and the Campbell Family Institute, where communication skills really do count

Contents

....

Preface

....

I want to make this book as practical and easy to use as possible. The object is to give you a set of useful guidelines to help you see your way through difficult situations. There are guidelines here that you can use for breaking bad news (the SPIKES strategy), for disclosing a medical error (CONES), for resolving conflict (HARD), and so on. In an ideal world, we would need only these few acronyms, but the others that you will find in this book are useful strategies to have in the "back of your mind" and may help you with some tasks, such as giving information to the patient.

I've organized the book in six chapters. Chapter 1 is a brief overview of the basic techniques that you will need (most of which you are probably using already). In particular, it focuses on the physical setting or physical context of the interview and how small things, such as getting your eyes on the same level as your patient's, can help.

Then I deal with what is undoubtedly the most important aspect of all difficult conversations: acknowledging your patient's feelings. As I'll show you, you do not have to experience your patient's feelings yourself (you are not required to "cry and bleed for every patient" and you probably couldn't feel the same emotions in most cases, anyway). However, you do need to respond to each "empathic opportunity" (i.e., respond to each major emotion that arises during your dialogue) with something that tells the patient that you recognize the emotion she or he is having right now and that you realize what prompted it. You do that by means of a fairly straightforward technique: the empathic response. It is a skill that you can learn quickly and use immediately. It is simple in practice, and the central point is to realize that our patients' emotions need to be acknowledged with a relatively straightforward statement.

In chapter 2, I set out the SPIKES protocol for sharing bad news, preceded by a definition of *bad news* and an overview of the many factors that make it so difficult for us when we have to break the news.

In chapter 3, I deal with those situations "when you have to tell"—of which probably the most difficult is the disclosing of medical error. Although nowadays there is almost universal acceptance of the principle that we *should* disclose any major errors, there are not yet any standardized strategies for *how* to do it. The CONES protocol may offer a useful framework and can be used in any situation in which you "have to tell," including informing a relative of the death of a patient, explaining adverse events, or explaining a sudden deterioration in a patient's condition.

In chapter 4, I share some practical ideas for dealing with escalation and conflict. As tensions mount, you may find the HARD strategy useful for decreasing the temperature and "the heat of the moment"—on both sides of the disagreement.

In chapter 5, I offer a few tips for giving information to a patient. Although this is a common type of interaction, it often isn't easy and is a common source of complaint and dissatisfaction. With the SAFER protocol, you have a chance to make information giving a bit more interactive and to make it easier for the patient to remember what you said.

In chapter 6, I suggest ways to approach some particularly awkward conversations, including requests for autopsy or organ donation, and describe some situations involving breaking bad news—examples of really difficult conversations.

In the conclusion, I outline a simple strategy for preparing yourself for a difficult interview. The ROSE protocol is a way of "getting it together" in the few seconds before you enter the room and start the conversation. As you will see throughout the book, this is a matter not of memorizing an infallible prefabricated script—there is no such thing, anyway—but of assembling in your mind the objectives of the conversation and the strategies that might help you achieve them.

Two other features of this book are worth mentioning. First, I have identified many "crossroads" to help you visualize your options at various points. Second, eight videotaped examples on the DVD that accompanies this book show you how these strategies can work in practice in a realistic time frame and clinical situation. It's worth discussing these two features in a little more detail.

The "Crossroads" Points: Options Available to You

Almost invariably, more options are available than you think (or fear). This book is all about making choices in an interview that are more likely to help it (and you) be seen as supportive. For that reason, you will find many examples of what can be termed *crossroads* points: moments when several options are available to you (even if you do not realize that at first).

To illustrate the format that I use throughout the text, here is an example of the options available in a situation that is relatively frequent and straightforward. A man presents to the emergency department with retrosternal chest pain. The ECG shows a small inferior MI. The patient asks what it shows, and you tell him.

He reacts sharply, opens his eyes wide, sits back against the pillows, and says, "A heart attack! Oh, no!" At that point, you could answer factually—a *direct or factual response*—and tell him that the chance of any serious immediate consequences is small. Or you could caution him not to overreact—a response that is likely to actually escalate tension, called an *escalation response*. Or you could ask him what particularly he was frightened of—an *open question*. Or you could acknowledge the emotion (or, rather, one of the emotions) with an *empathic response* (which I describe in detail in chapter 1 and refer to often thereafter).

To make it easier for you to visualize the options, I will express them in the following format, summarizing the situation and the patient's (or family's) reaction and setting out some of the choices that you have.

➤ *Situation:*
The patient has had an episode of retrosternal chest pain. The ECG shows a small inferior MI. You tell the patient that he has had a small heart attack.

> *The Patient Says:*
> "A heart attack! Oh, no!"
> *You Can Choose from:*
> —*Direct or Factual Response:*
> "I did say it was a *small* heart attack."
> —*Escalationary or Judgmental Response:*
> "There's no need to panic, you know."

—*Open Question:*
   "Tell me what's going through your mind."
—*Empathic Response:*
   "This is obviously a big shock."

As you can see, in each of the four categories is one example of that type of response. And that is significant: the exact words and phrasing you use in a particular approach are not crucial, but the approach you choose is important. For example, there are probably dozens of empathic responses that you could use (e.g., "I realize you're shocked" or "Clearly, that's distressing" or "I can see that's upsetting" or, more colloquially, "That's obviously not what you wanted to hear"). Any of those will do. They are all equally effective—and they are all different from saying something like, "There's no need to panic, you know."

In most situations, empathic responses are the ones that are most likely to help you—by which I mean they are most likely to help you help the patient. Using an open question is rarely wrong, however. You can think of an empathic response as a valuable way of dealing with an emotion when you can see clearly what the emotion is, and an open question as a useful "range-finder" to help you determine the main emotion the patient is experiencing when you are not sure. For that reason, when you see the "crossroads" throughout this book, you can think of the last two responses as more useful than the first two.

Yes, But How? One Example Is Worth a Thousand Words

As a further illustration of these techniques, you can look at the accompanying DVD. In the scenarios on the DVD, you will see several clinical situations in which an actor (a standardized patient) portrays the patient and I portray the physician using one of the protocols to deal with the situation.

All of the scenarios on the DVD are unscripted and unrehearsed: they are spontaneous. In each case, the standardized patient knew the medical facts of the condition that he or she was representing but was not instructed as to what to say or how to respond. I must tell you that the actors were so good at role-playing that within a few seconds of the start of each scenario, I had completely forgotten that they were actors, and I responded as I would to an actual patient.

In many ways, those scenarios are almost the equivalent of an apprenticeship in communication skills. They show you how these things can work out in practice and are helpful if you cannot witness one of those interviews for yourself. (In real life, such situations happen at unpredictable times, and often the patient doesn't want additional people present.)

Just as we learned many of the rules of clinical examination by example, from watching our trainers in action, so these videotaped scenarios illustrate how the steps of a protocol may lead logically from one to the next. You don't have to (and shouldn't try to) use the same words or phrases as those in the scenarios, but you can see how the approach works in real life (or at least a close simulation of real life). What you will see in the scenarios on the DVD are examples of the *strategies* in action; you don't need to worry too much about the exact script.

Practical Plans for Difficult Conversations in Medicine

Prescribing the Doctor as Part of the Treatment

The Doctor as Part of the Treatment

As a doctor, you are a vital component of the treatment that you offer to your patient. To put it simply, the objective of this book is to help you—as a health care professional—to enhance and augment your communication skills and hence reinforce a crucial component of the treatment of the patient.

Let me explain in a bit more detail. The relationship between the patient and the professional can be boiled down to two basic equations:

1. Patient = Disease + Person

and

2. Treatment = Medication* + Health Care Professional

   (* or surgery or therapy or other procedure)

It is worthwhile examining those two key principles for a moment.

First, as we all know, a patient is not defined totally and solely by the medical condition that she or he has. For instance, imagine two patients who have brittle diabetes, each with a daily insulin requirement of eighty units. If one patient is slightly obsessive, careful about her diet, and attentive to her glucose monitoring, it is likely that her HbA_1C and her performance in terms of visual, renal, and cardiovascular function might be near normal. If the other patient happens to be an entrepreneurial type and an owner of a bar and drinks alcohol frequently for the sake of encouraging his clientele and also has a less-attentive attitude to his health and to his insulin injections, it might not be surprising if his HbA$_1$C is high and his retinal, renal, and cardiovascular complications problematic. In these two cases, the "disease" part of the equation is nearly the same, but because the "person" is different, the health outcomes for the two patients will be different.

The second of those two equations is also important. You, as a physician or other health care professional, are not totally and solely defined by the interventions (the medications, surgery, procedures, etc.) that you administer to your patient. Just as the patient is not synonymous with the disease, you are not defined by the intervention.

When you prescribe, let's say, an antihypertensive medication for a patient who has hypertension, the effect on the diastolic pressure does not depend solely on the medication that you choose: it also depends on the way in which you elicited the history, how you assessed the impact of the diagnosis on the patient (for example, the degree of anxiety or absence of it), and dozens of other factors contributing to your relationship with the "person" part of the patient. Whether the patient takes the medication regularly—and hence its effectiveness—will depend to some extent on the process that has gone on between you, as will the patient's perception of the illness, the treatment, the concept of health, and so on. A beta-blocker prescribed by you is not the same treatment as the identical beta-blocker prescribed by another physician. Whether the patient decides to take it regularly and how the patient feels about it, its effect, and its side effects depends on you as well as on the pharmacology of the drug.

Your treatment and its effect on the "disease + person" is therefore a combination of what you do and how you do it. This book will help you to improve "how you do it."

As you are going to see in this book, that part of professional behavior is not as nebulous or mystical (nor as demanding in terms of time and effort) as you might fear. Communication strategies and approaches can be used that greatly improve the situation. Furthermore, these strategies and protocols can be used in the same way in which we use standardized approaches to auscultation or assessing limb paralysis. After a time, they become your usual and accustomed way of doing a clinical examination; in the same way, after a time these strategies can become your usual and accustomed way of having difficult conversations. They are not scripts, but they are strategies, and they work.

As with all aspects of clinical interactions, some subjective factors are involved, but even so, nothing is mysterious or mystical about communication. It is a matter of tuition rather than intuition. The principles of the approach and the *modus operandi* can be described plainly and simply and can be learned in the same way that you learned how to palpate the abdomen. And like all aspects of taking a history and performing an examination, this is the foundation of the doctor-patient relationship and will be helpful to both parties.

Dealing with communication in the same way as other aspects of clinical interaction makes this book a little unusual. Most standard textbooks of medicine and almost all of our training courses (appropriately) focus on "disease-doctoring"—on examining and perfecting the diagnosis and treatment of the myriad conditions that cause problems. Much less of our time and training has, until recently, been devoted to "person-doctoring"—even though we all acknowledge that this makes a great deal of difference to the doctor-patient relationship and thus to the success of (and compliance with) our treatment.

This book is a systematic approach to improving "person-doctoring." It is an attempt to outline the science of the art of clinical practice and to help you use your own communication as part of your treatment of the patient. In other words, I focus on the factors that facilitate the activity of "prescribing the doctor."

I'd like to make one other reassuring point: communication skills are in many ways like driving skills. With a bit of tuition and practice, we can all become reasonable (and reasonably safe) drivers. Almost all of us will be able at some point to pass a driving test. Of course, some people seem to be natural drivers, to have an almost innate understanding of the spatial relationships of cars on the road and to be almost unerring in their judgment and decision making. (I'm not one of those people, by the way.) The same is true of communication skills: some people are almost "naturals" at communicating. (I'm not one of those people either; I had to learn and practice all the techniques that I discuss here to be able to do the tasks that I describe.) Even if you think you are near the bottom of this scale in terms of natural communicating abilities, that doesn't matter. The skills that I describe in this book are all learnable, so almost anyone—however innately clumsy he or she may think he or she is—can bring him- or herself up to the average standard (which means that average standard will rise, as everyone in the bottom half moves up toward the middle).

So do not be daunted. All of these techniques—including the examples on the accompanying DVD—are learnable. They can be acquired and practiced until they gradually become part of the way you conduct your clinical practice.

The Hourglass

At this point, you might be thinking, "That's all very well, but there simply isn't time for all this stuff." A reasonable thought—but not correct. There *is* time for this because strategies and approaches to difficult situations will, in the end, save you time (rather than costing you time) and increase your efficiency.

In daily practice, we are all aware that time is short. Furthermore, while the clock is ticking, we are also painfully aware of the vast number of items that we are supposed to discuss with our patients. That is inevitable because we and our patients have a lot of issues that we want to address. The catalogue of topics accumulates on both sides of the discussion. On our side are the medical management topics and care plans; on the patient's side are the symptoms, worries, and concerns.

Of course, the accumulation of issues begins long before the moment in which we meet with the patient. Patients come to the clinic or onto the ward with—naturally—a large number of fears and concerns: the diagnosis, the prognosis, the treatment, the situation at home or at work, and dozens more. At the same time, on our side of the discussion we have an enormous amount to think about: the best management plan, the chances of response, the side effects and sequelae of treatment, and then explaining all of this to the patient, along with many other issues. Somehow, we have to make a credible effort in sorting all this out in a short time.

Perhaps the best model for conceptualizing the pressure created by the large number of items to be processed during the brief clinician-patient meeting is the image of the hourglass—and its rate-limiting middle constriction that defines it. The time we spend with our patients is comparable to the bottleneck in the hourglass—with an added complication: in clinical interviews there is not only a traffic problem but also an organizational

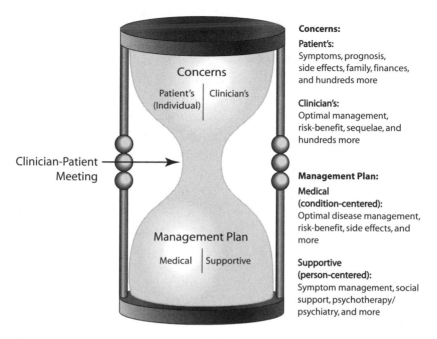

Concerns:

Patient's:
Symptoms, prognosis, side effects, family, finances, and hundreds more

Clinician's:
Optimal management, risk-benefit, sequelae, and hundreds more

Management Plan:

Medical (condition-centered):
Optimal disease management, risk-benefit, side effects, and more

Supportive (person-centered):
Symptom management, social support, psychotherapy/psychiatry, and more

The Hourglass

problem. We cannot simply allow the issues to trickle passively through like the sand in the hourglass; we also have to process them and combine our interventions into a plan of care that will meet, as far as is possible, the medical situation and provide support for the patient. (See figure.)

Furthermore, even approaching those "nondisease" aspects of the situation is often daunting. To put it frankly, many of us are anxious about what we might start if we open a discussion about the patient's concerns or fears. If we even mention the subject of psychosocial needs, will we open a Pandora's box? If we ask about anxieties and the patient is, at that particular moment, not very worried, will we then create anxieties? Will the patient minimize the extent of the symptoms, perhaps causing us to miss an importance diagnosis? Or exaggerate them, prompting unhelpful investigations?

Then, having raised an issue and a concern, what are we expected to do about it? What can we do about it? Aren't we supposed to have all the answers?

For all of these reasons, we clinicians are often reluctant to open discussions of difficult topics. Fortunately, there are approaches and strategies that can help, as you shall see.

The objective of this book, then, is to provide some of the answers and some ways of improving our communication so that we can improve the flow through that constriction in the hourglass—to make the clinician-patient time more efficient and to focus more effectively on dealing with the medical condition and with the patient's concerns.

All of the techniques in this book are practical ways of increasing the capacity and efficiency of the bottleneck in the hourglass—and it all depends on communication. After all, during the clinician-patient meeting, the only tool available to you at that moment is communication, which is why any tips and guidelines have to be practical and have to work in a busy clinic with real patients in real time.

This book sets out strategies or approaches to difficult situations. It provides guidelines, not mandatory orders or prefabricated solutions. It is not a set of scripts or prefabricated phrases that will solve the problem. No such entities exist, anyway: no magical formulaic phrases can be used universally to remedy a particular type of difficult situation.

But there are guidelines, and there are hints and tips. What you will find here are some examples and some hints as to what you might say, but they are no more than illustrations; they are not mandatory statements or prescribed "correct" phrases. They will show you some of the many possible ways of expressing a thought and—if they seem to work for you—will make you feel that the task can be done and that there are ways of approaching a difficult moment, when otherwise you might have been feeling beleaguered and directionless. By the time you've gone through the various strategies here, you will want to use your own words and phrasings, and that is exactly the way it should be.

In the Heat of the Moment: Why Strategies Are Useful

If this book works for you, you will find ways of continuing conversations at moments when (as happens to all of us!) your immediate thought might otherwise have been, "I have no idea what to say now." To put it bluntly, when an interview is becoming tense, it is difficult to remember anything at all, even logical and helpful hints and tips. In the heat of the moment, our minds are likely to go almost blank.

For that reason, almost every subspecialty has its own strategies, acronyms, and aide-mémoires to help physicians deal with a clinical problem such as diabetic keto-acidosis, cardiac arrest, or coma. Doctor-patient communication is no different. When things are difficult and awkward, we need a simple strategy so that we can proceed with a constructive approach at the moment when we are (probably) feeling that we have no idea of what to say or how to approach the topic. Just as the A-B-C-D-E acronym for resuscitation after cardiac arrest (Airway, Breathing, Cardiac compression, Drugs, Electricity) is a useful way of dealing with that emergency and quelling the anxieties that we all feel for the first few times, so the acronyms that you will find here are a framework by which you can remember a logical sequence of steps at a time when you are probably having difficulty remembering anything.

After a time, you will find that when you have to share bad news, the SPIKES strategy comes readily to mind, and the same is true for the CONES strategy for disclosing error, the HARD approach to resolving conflict, and so on. The text explains what each of the steps involves, and on the enclosed DVD you will find demonstrations of how these approaches work in real (or at least realistically simulated!) clinical practice.

CHAPTER ONE

Some "Can't Go Wrong" Tips

Being a good communicator is an acquired skill (not an inborn gift)

1.1. Starting Off Well: Nonverbal Communication and Body Language

Communication Techniques Are Like Table Manners

Although the following points might appear at first to be overly fussy and to deal with matters too small to deserve your attention, they are not. In many ways, these little tricks are comparable to good table manners. It might seem strict for us to tell our children that they shouldn't chew with their mouths open or wave their forks above their heads, but, as we know, grown people who do those things are perceived as rather crass and crude.

It is the same with the following few simple rules of body language and nonverbal communication. If you do not pay any attention to at least some of these points, the other person will think of you as uninterested in effective communication and will be less forthcoming.

Furthermore, there is some positive reinforcement for you. Once you see the benefit of good communication techniques on your clinical interactions, it will make you feel more confident, and your patient will perceive that increase in confidence and comfort as increased competence. In other words, there is a secondary gain for you in all of these.

The opposite also applies. If you have no idea how to handle the breaking of bad news, you will try to avoid it, which makes it even worse the next time the situation arises.

So, for all these reasons, it is worth your acquiring a few basic techniques (if you are not using them already—and if you are, please skip the next section).

Some Useful Basic Tips

1. THE GREETING

I recommend shaking hands with the patient as you come into the room to meet him or her (or as the patient comes into the room to meet you). Of course, this is a matter of personal style and choice, but I think it almost always starts things off well. (There is also a public health matter here: I do not shake hands if I have a cold and during the flu season, and I tell the patient that. Also I make sure I wash/disinfect my hands before and after examining the patient.)

If you haven't met the patient before, use the person's name ("Hello. Are you Mr. Thompson?"). I know it sounds silly, but twice in my career I used the patient's name at the start of the interview—and several times during the interview—only to find later that it wasn't Mr. Thompson that I'd been talking to at all but another patient entirely. So even a proper introduction isn't an infallible guarantee. Then, having established who *the patient* is, the next step is to establish who *you* are. Tell the patient your name (I show my ID badge as well)—sometimes the patient is expecting a different doctor—and say, in a couple of words, what you do.

These points about introduction and greeting are mostly a matter of courtesy, but they also set the frame for the whole interview. It is *always* helpful that the patient thinks of you as courteous.

2. GET YOUR EYES ON THE SAME LEVEL AS THE OTHER PERSON'S

This may be the most important tip in organizing a good "setup" for the interview. It makes a big difference if your eyes are on the same level as the patient's. This almost always means that you have to sit down (if the patient is sitting down). I cannot overemphasize the value of this maneuver. If you stay standing when the patient is seated, the patient will feel uncomfortable and will probably perceive you as not being supportive (and will tell friends that). So sit down, and if the patient happens to be short, you can simply hunch over or slouch a little so that you are on each other's eye level.

3. TRY TO LOOK RELAXED

In most of the situations that I shall be discussing, you will probably not be feeling relaxed. That goes with the territory. The secret (as every psychiatrist and psychotherapist knows) it to try to look relaxed, calm, and in control of the situation, even if you don't feel that way.

The easiest way of doing this is to adopt a body posture often called "the neutral body posture." Most psychiatrists and psychotherapists use it, and all you do is to put your feet flat on the floor with your ankles together and your knees together, then put your hands palm down on your lap. If you are sitting at a desk with the patient's chart, then just rest your hands on the table edge.

There are two important points about this body posture. First, you are avoiding the body signals of anxiety, fidgeting, defensiveness, etc. By adopting this simple posture, you are basically telling the patient that you are "open for business." Second, after you have done this a few times, it starts making you feel more relaxed. Simply knowing what to do and being comfortable doing it will move you toward a more helpful frame of mind.

4. HAVE LESS THAN FOUR FEET OF SPACE BETWEEN YOU

Curiously enough, there is no universal "best buy" for the amount of space between you and your patient. In general terms, in Western cultures and in urban areas, it is expected that people should be about three feet away from each other, and some studies show that about two feet is usually satisfactory. In rural areas, that distance is usually bigger. Also, there are gender differences: what is acceptable in female-female conversation may seem somewhat predatory in a male-female interview. In general, it is almost always satisfactory to have the distance between you less than four feet, and about three feet is usually good.

Another point that I recommend is that you sit across the corner of the desk from the patient rather than across the width of the table. There is a small amount of evidence supporting this,[1] but I have found that in every clinic where I have worked, the simple placement of the patient's chair at the side of the desk (rather than on the opposite side) makes the atmosphere feel more conducive to a useful discussion.

5. LEAN FORWARD

Having greeted the other person and seated yourself in a good position, then lean forward. There are studies showing that patients interpret the doctor's leaning forward as a sign that she or he is interested.[2] This simple action will help set you up as being good at "people-doctoring."

6. SHOW THAT YOU ARE IN "LISTENING MODE"

A vast number of techniques can be used to facilitate an interview. Of these, I would single out two really useful ones: *silence* (when the patient is talking) and *repetition* (meaning that your first sentence after the patient has spoken contains one or two key words from the patient's last sentence).

Silence requires a lot of effort. One famous study showed that medics tend to interrupt their patients after an average of eighteen seconds.[3] Now that study was rather strict in that if the doctor said, "Tell me more," that counted as an interruption; nevertheless, it was interesting to note that the vast proportion of patients finished what they were saying by two minutes, anyway. I find it also helps to make sure that while you are listening, you have your mouth closed (thus avoiding sending an inadvertent signal that you are waiting to interrupt).

It also helps to repeat a word or two from what the patient says. If you repeat a word with a rising intonation—as in the following example—it facilitates the conversation and helps you find out more accurately what the patient means.

Patient: I'm fed up with those medications!
Doctor: Fed up?
Patient: Yeah. The side effects.
Doctor: Side effects?
Patient: I mean, they make me feel so lousy.
Doctor: Lousy?
Patient: Dizzy. You know, woozy. Even spacey sometimes.

Each time the doctor repeats a word, he or she basically invites the patient to expand on the previous statement (when the doctor might initially have no idea what the issue is). Furthermore, the doctor gains a moment or two to focus on the crux of what the patient is saying.

7. BE READY TO SMILE

Smiling is a matter of personal style and choice, but it rarely does harm! If you do smile, try to smile "with your whole face," not just with your mouth. Apparently, people can distinguish easily between a "whole-face" smile, which is interpreted as a genuine sign of goodwill, and a "lips-only" smile, which is usually interpreted as insincere or even as a snarl.

TABLE 1.1 *A Few Basic Tips*

Technique	Central Feature	Notes
Greeting	Use the person's name.	A simple way of establishing the "person" as well as the "problem"
Introduce yourself	Briefly say who you are and what you do.	Merely courteous
Shake hands	Make actual contact.	Don't do that if you have a cold.
Sit down!	Bring your eyes to the same level as the other person's.	Essential
Don't be too far away	Have less than four feet of space between you.	The optimal distance varies with gender and culture, but three feet is rarely wrong.
Adopt a neutral body posture	Look relaxed, or at least not too anxious or irritated.	Even if you don't feel relaxed (and most of us don't at these times), try to adopt the neutral body posture and look relaxed.
Lean forward	Don't sit back all the way against the chair.	Studies show that patients recognize this as a sign of being interested in them.
Be ready to smile	Smiling may not be your usual "thing," but it helps if you can manage it.	If you do smile, try to "smile with your whole face."
Switch on your listening skills	Silence and repetition	Consciously maintain silence as the patient starts talking. Then in your first sentence of response use a word or phrase from the patient's last sentence.

This may involve the contraction of the zygomatic major muscle, which influences the interpretation of the smile.[4]

The few straightforward techniques listed in table 1.1 will help you set up the interview well. However, the most important communication technique is the one you use to acknowledge the emotional content of the interview. The simplest and most straightforward way of doing that is called the empathic response, which is the subject of the next section.

1.2. The Empathic Response: The Most Useful Communication Technique of All

The empathic response is the simplest and most direct way of acknowledging another person's emotion. It basically allows you to tell the other person that you have seen and observed some of the feelings that he or she is experiencing. It does not abolish or fix or "cure" those emotions, nor does it imply that you are experiencing the same emotion that the other person is feeling (which is impossible, anyway). It just tells the other person that you are paying attention to the emotional component of the dialogue. It is without doubt the most useful communication technique for any difficult conversation.

The empathic response consists of three steps:

STEP 1: IDENTIFY ONE OF THE EMOTIONS

Most of us experience a mixture of several emotions at the same time. For example, on hearing a piece of bad news, we may feel some fear, some anger, and some disappointment, and we might also have difficulty comprehending it (disbelief) or even want to shut out the news (denial). All of those emotions might coexist behind a shocked "Oh, no!"

So when the patient shows an emotional response (such as "Oh, no!"), you simply need to decide on *one* of the emotions that you can see. (And the fact that you can see the emotional expression clearly shows that it is a "big" experience, something the patient feels intensely and deeply.)

Having fixed on one of the emotions in the mixture, name it (in your own mind). Say to yourself, "This patient is clearly shocked," or "He's angry now," or "She's having difficulty believing what I just said." Don't be afraid of using words with wide, all-inclusive meanings, such as *shock* or *distress* or *upset* and so on.

STEP 2: IDENTIFY THE CAUSE OF THE EMOTION

Usually the cause of the emotion is the piece of news that you have just given or the topic that one of you has just raised. That is all you need. You don't need to perform some miracle of psychoanalysis ("This man is upset because he now sees his career and relationships as total failures and is doubtful that he can recreate his lost youth"). All you need do in step 2 is to pinpoint the immediate cause of the emotional reaction; often it will be something that you have just said.

STEP 3: RESPOND IN A WAY THAT SHOWS YOU HAVE MADE THE CONNECTION BETWEEN STEPS 1 AND 2

Tell the patient that you have observed his or her feelings and that you are aware of what evoked that emotion. Empathic responses (and there are hundreds, of course!) are usually in the form of "Clearly, that's a major shock," or "You are obviously upset by this," or "I realize that this is awful for you," or "This is difficult to take in, isn't it?"

When you respond to a patient's feelings with an empathic response, you achieve three objectives simultaneously:

1. *You legitimize that person's feelings.* You are telling the patient that the emotion he or she is experiencing *is* an understandable response to the situation. In doing that, you are showing that you are not making a judgment about the emotion.

2. *You are telling the person that it is permissible to discuss those feelings.* You are demonstrating that feelings are legitimate items on the agenda between the two of you. In the words of the cliché: "We can talk about this."

3. *You change the subject.* For that moment, you are not talking about the infarct or the hypertension or the bowel cancer; you are talking about how the person *feels* at this moment in response to that information.

In other words, you are showing the patient that you have noted his or her feelings, however briefly, and are including those emotions as part of your overall approach to the clinical situation.

So the empathic response is not a standard formula of words—it's not a catchphrase or motto—it is a response that identifies, addresses, and acknowledges the expressed emotion.

Table 1.2 shows some examples of different ways you could respond to the patient I mentioned in the preface—the man who said, "A heart attack! Oh, no!" The left side of the table shows responses that address the emotion (and are therefore empathic responses), and the right side shows ones that don't.

TABLE 1.2

Empathic Responses These address and express the emotion.	Other Responses These do not address the emotion.
"Clearly, this is a big shock."	"It's not *that* bad."
"This seems very scary, doesn't it?"	"We'll get you up to the CCU right away."
"That's obviously awful for you."	"It's a treatable situation."
"I can see this is upsetting for you."	"Don't make it worse for yourself."
"I know that's not what you wanted to hear."	"There's no need to panic about this."
"You seem shocked by this news."	"Please settle down."
"That's obviously a big surprise and shock."	"You'll be feeling much better soon."
	"It's only a *small* heart attack, you know."

Right now, as you read this, you might be thinking, "This is not a very big deal." But it is. Although the empathic response takes only a few seconds, it demonstrates to the patient that you are aware of the "person" part of the "illness + person" side of the equation. If you *don't* acknowledge (however briefly) the patient's feelings, you will be perceived as being insensitive (patients often use the words *cold* and even *cruel*).

The empathic response is a technique that is the most valuable adjunct to your plan of medical management.

So What's the Difficulty?

There is just one further point to make about the empathic response: it is very different from our usual, accustomed, and learned responses to medical symptoms. If a patient says, "I've had a pain in my abdomen for about three hours," our first thoughts are probably, "Could this be appendicitis?" or "Is this an acute abdomen (i.e., a surgical emergency)?" These instant reactions are entirely appropriate: appropriately, we are not accustomed to responding simply by saying something like "This must be very unpleasant for you." We are trained—correctly—to assess and sift and evaluate what we hear from our patients. At first sight, therefore, you might think that an empathic response is the opposite of—or even contradictory to—that critical analysis of the patient's symptoms. It is not; rather, it is *complementary* to your handling of the medical situation. You need to do both things: to analyze and manage the clinical problem and to acknowledge the emotions that arise from it. It is not difficult to achieve those two objectives at the same time.

It is worth emphasizing that nothing in the empathic response—or in the whole of this book—negates our usual medical process for assessing and dealing with the patient's medical condition. The empathic response is an *adjunct*: it is a simple way of acknowledging how the patient is feeling when those feelings are running high. It would be fair to say that acknowledging the patient's emotions is the main difference between the "treatment" (as a one-dimensional medical intervention) and the "doctor" (as a combination of the treatment and a responding individual).

Are Doctors Good at This?

Unfortunately, some recent studies have shown that physicians are not very good at responding to emotions in clinical practice. In one such study, the investigators videotaped (with full consent) conversations between cancer patients and their oncologists.[5] The videotapes were then rigorously coded to identify moments at which the patient said something that indicated a major emotion (for example, "I've got nothing to look forward to"). Approximately four hundred of these moments—termed "empathic opportunities"—were identified. Of those four hundred emotional signals, the oncologists responded by exploring the emotion in only 22 percent. In 76 percent of the situations, the oncologists responded with a direct change in the management plan or restatement of fact (responses that were labeled—perhaps inelegantly—as "terminators").

A further study described a similar study of lung cancer patients (as opposed to patients who had any type of cancer, as in the first study). With lung cancer patients, the results were even worse: the oncologists responded to the emotional cue in only 11 percent of cases.[6]

So the answer to the question, "Are doctors good at this?" is "Unfortunately no, we're not good at this."

There are many reasons for this lack. Predominantly, we are chosen for medical school for our ability in problem management and technical skills, and as we progress through our training, those demonstrable and testable skills are the main focus of our training. As I've said above, it is entirely appropriate that we are taught how to manage diabetic keto-acidosis or hypercalcemia or any of the thousands of medical conditions that we might encounter, but inadvertently during the process of our learning all that, the relatively straightforward skills of communication somehow get pushed aside.

That doctors are demonstrably poor at responding to emotional factors is a remediable problem (and all the techniques described in this book are part of the remedy). Dealing with emotional issues and "person-doctoring" are simply *additional* skills that can, should, and must be incorporated into our everyday clinical practice, alongside all of the technical knowledge and diagnostic and problem-solving abilities. Our patients clearly need us to respond to emotional factors, and it has been shown in many studies that we can learn to meet those needs.[7]

Your Own Emotions

Another important feature of the empathic response is that you can use it to acknowledge your own feelings.

If you happen to be feeling frustrated with a patient who wants to try, let's say, herbal remedies for a bacterial pneumonia, it would be far more constructive for you to make an empathic response to your own feelings and to say something like, "I'm getting worried that you can't accept the dangers of this pneumonia" rather than exploding with, "Will you shut up about your damned herbal stuff!"

In framing an empathic response to your own emotions, you are effectively—and helpfully—stating an objective observation of your own subjective feelings. In other words, you are *explaining* your feelings rather than *exhibiting* them, and *describing* them rather than *displaying* them. It may not seem a big difference, but in practice it is. Even if you don't know what to say, you are better off saying, "I don't know what to say" rather than becoming silent and being perceived as sullen.

Kindergarten teachers are fond of saying to agitated children, "Use your words." Making an empathic response is one way of doing precisely that.

1.3. Time Management

As I said in the analogy of the hourglass, time is a resource that is always scarce.

There is some good evidence showing that the time spent in an interview has virtually no correlation with the satisfaction felt by the patient (or the parents of the patient in pediatric practice[8]). You can spend three hours and still not touch on the crux of the problem, and you can spend eight minutes and get right to the heart of the matter. In the scenarios on the DVD, I concentrated particularly on covering the ground in less than fifteen minutes per interview. Even though the issues were often difficult—medical error, news of a death, and recurrence of bowel cancer, among others—I felt it important to imagine that the interview was taking place in a realistic and realizable time frame; rarely do we have much longer than fifteen minutes. There are a few exceptions; for example, I would suggest that explanation of a clinical trial and recruiting a patient into it requires an additional fifteen minutes (on average). But in all the video scenarios that I recorded (there are about sixty of them in total on the two sets of CD-ROMs[9]), as well as in the eight samples of them that are included on the DVD that comes with this book, I consciously set myself a time limit of fifteen minutes for each interview. So these communication tasks can be completed within a time frame appropriate to busy clinical practice.

You Are Allowed to Call "Time"

As I said in the analogy of the hourglass, our time is precious. Fortunately, we are allowed to say that!

The normal social rules of time management include giving notice of the approach of the end of the interview. The secret is to make that statement near the end of the interview, not near the beginning, and to make it as unemotionally and unhurriedly as possible.

This technique improves with practice, but it is, of course, the everyday practice of everybody involved in psychotherapy and every discipline in which discussion is the main therapeutic modality.

1.4. Summary: A Good Aim for All Interviews Is "Sensitive Decisiveness"

The empathic response—the central technique of "person-doctoring"—is a crucial adjunct to medical management and not a substitute for it. Our patients want us to respond to the human side of their situation, and the empathic response is of major value in achieving that. However, they also want—and expect—us to do our best to fix their medical problem.

Perhaps the best phrase to embrace both of those objectives is "sensitive decisiveness." We have to make up our minds and decide on a plan of management for the patient's medical problem *and* we have to show that we are aware of the patient's feelings (when they are intense) at the same time. (Fortunately, we can do both during one interaction, as you will see throughout this book.)

Patients—often appropriately—equate decisiveness with expertise. They expect us to be aware of the best options in handling their medical situation and to be able to state that. Even when there are two equally appropriate options (say, in the initial management of a small breast cancer with either lumpectomy followed by radiation or simple mastectomy), our patients can justifiably expect us to say something like, "Medically speaking, in situations like this, there is no difference in terms of outcome, so your own preferences are important." It is possible to express that choice in a normal and decisive manner and still acknowledge that this particular patient might have strong personal preferences for one form of treatment rather than the other. Acknowledging the patient's emotions does not in any way undermine the medical management. Sensitive decisiveness is a response that covers both objectives, without detracting from either.

The SPIKES Protocol for Breaking Bad News

		Topics covered in this chapter
S	**S**etting and **S**tarting	Sit down, body language, eye contact, touch. Open questions, silence, and repetition.
P	**P**erception	Assess what the patient knows or suspects. Listen to vocabulary and comprehension.
I	**I**nvitation	Obtain permission to share knowledge or set an agenda.
K	**K**nowledge	Align with the patient's understanding, use plain language, give information in small chunks.
E	**E**motions	Acknowledge major emotions as they arise.
S	**S**trategy and **S**ummary	Set out a plan of medical management. Close with précis, any questions, and contract for next contact.

CHAPTER TWO

Breaking Bad News

The SPIKES Protocol

....

Before you tell, ask

2.1. A Definition of Bad News: Two Crucial Components

....

The most important feature of bad news is that it lowers the patient's *expectations of the future.* In other words, bad news can be defined as any new information that seriously and adversely alters the patient's expectations of the future.[1]

This definition not only highlights the most challenging and upsetting aspect of the bad news but also offers us a logical approach to the process of sharing it with the patient.

This definition implies that you have no idea how bad the bad news is—in other words, you have no idea of the *impact* of what you are about to discuss—until you find out what the patient already knows or suspects about the situation. To put it in the form of a simple motto: "Before you tell, ask." That straightforward principle is the central idea of the SPIKES protocol.

As you go through the six steps of the SPIKES protocol, you will see that there are two main issues to be dealt with simultaneously: (1) the *medical facts* and (2) the *patient's emotional responses* to those facts. With the SPIKES protocol—particularly with the use of the empathic response when strong emotions are expressed—you can deal with both of these issues during the interview, and you can be supportive and helpful to the patient, even though you are the one imparting the bad news. To put it another way, even though the message is unpleasant, you can still be a valuable messenger. Let's start by briefly summarizing why the task of the messenger is so difficult.

2.2. Why Breaking Bad News Is So Difficult

Several factors make breaking bad news difficult. It is not simply due to the fact that the news itself is bad. There are other aspects to it, and it is worth spending a moment looking at the components of the difficulty that we all face when we break bad news.

Basically, you can think of these difficulties under eight headings.

1. BLAMING THE MESSENGER

Bad news, as defined above, is always accompanied by disappointment. Much of the distress, of course, is caused by the news itself and its implications. Often, though, the messenger takes some of the blame. That is not necessarily the fault of the messenger's manner of transmitting the message; it is simply a human mechanism for coping with bad news. The process is often called "personification," and it means "blaming the messenger for the message." It is a human reaction that is as old as human history; in Egyptian and Roman civilizations, it was customary to execute the messenger if he brought bad news.

Almost all of us currently perform some type of personification at various points in our daily lives. For example, think how we all tend to react when we come back to our car and find an officer writing out a parking ticket. Even though our real anger is with the bureaucracy of the parking office and with our own miscalculation in parking illegally when we thought it would go unnoticed, it is easy for us to transfer that anger onto the officer himself, and to dislike the air of smugness and satisfaction that this particular officer seems to be exuding, and to resent his arbitrary decision to write the ticket instead of giving us a couple of extra minutes! Few of us habitually respond to that situation by saying something like, "Ah! I deserved that ticket for parking there, officer. Thanks for teaching me a lesson." Sainthood awaits anyone who responds like that every time.

So we all, in everyday life, may experience these small flashes of irritation and may divert them partly—whether verbally or silently—toward the messenger. Personification is not a new or alien type of reaction; it is something we are all familiar with. Furthermore, the symbols of the messenger's role or job make it even easier to shift the blame. Because the officer is wearing the uniform of the parking ticket office, we may feel slightly more justified in railing against the nameless and faceless bureaucracy of that office, and we may feel that we are not *really* shouting at Officer Smith, the father of two children, who is just doing his job, and so on.

The mechanism by which this occurs with the officer and the ticket is the same mechanism that operates between the patient and us in the clinic. The symbols of our role, the badges of office that we display as health care professionals, make this blaming process easier—whether the symbols are visible or behavioral. Whether we are wearing a lab coat or not, there are many reminders and emblems of our role, underlying many aspects of the way we talk and the way we behave. These distinguishing features are the things that allow us every day to transgress normal social boundaries when we ask direct personal questions and examine the patient. Hence, when it comes to breaking bad news, these same distinguishing features act like the officer's uniform and inadvertently provide a way of making it easier for the patient to personify the bad news and to blame us as messengers, even if we are doing an almost faultless job in delivering the message.

In fact, the more control we exert over the patient's situation—as we organize the tests and the treatment and so on—the greater we make this effect. The more control we appear to have, the more we line ourselves up to be blamed when things do not go well.

I am not saying that we should do things differently—we cannot and should not abrogate responsibility for managing our patients' care—but we do need to be aware that along with the control over events comes the risk of being blamed. Merely realizing that this responsibility is one source of being blamed will help us cope with it.

2. STRONG EMOTIONS

We are often aware that bad news may trigger a big emotional reaction in the patient. Most of us in the nonpsychiatric specialties have not had a great deal of training in handling emotion, so we find the prospect of dealing with this emotional turbulence difficult. In fact, the more accomplished we are in our own field, the more difficult it is to accept that we have not been shown how to do this apparently simple task of dealing with a patient who is crying or shouting or who remains completely silent. In general, we do not relish having to do something at which we feel relatively unskilled, so this reluctance is another factor that causes us to flinch mentally as we come to impart bad news.

If such discomfort is a major factor in your own situation, you will be relieved to know that this book's central purpose is to explain how emotions can be dealt with and acknowledged in a fairly straightforward fashion and that those techniques can be acquired like any other clinical skill.

3. FEELINGS IN SYMPATHY

Another factor that makes breaking bad news difficult is that we may experience feelings similar to the disappointment or pain our patient experiences when hearing the news. The feelings that we experience as echoes or resonances of the other person's feelings are called "feelings in sympathy," and the extent to which we, as professionals, have these feelings varies widely. Some of us experience those feelings rarely and some not at all. In itself, this doesn't matter. It matters only if you happen to be the kind of person who does have feelings in sympathy often or intensely: if you do, you will find breaking bad news even more painful.

4. FEELINGS OF PROFESSIONAL FAILURE

As health care professionals, we want to fix our patients' problems and we enjoy doing it. If the bad news that we impart includes problems that are incurable or unfixable, we are likely to feel a sense of professional failure, which may spill over into a sense of personal inadequacy.

Even if we know that we have used the best available treatment for this patient's condition, there still lurks a vague and unspoken fear that somewhere, some other physician may have a miraculous cure for exactly this problem.

This vague professional queasiness is another factor that makes discussions of conditions for which there is no major medical treatment even more uncomfortable.

5. MEDICOLEGAL FACTORS

Until recently, the specter of medicolegal (and financial) complications loomed large in discussions about bad news. It was often difficult, particularly in the United States, to discuss freely, for example, a poor prognosis. At times it seemed that, for any adverse medical event, even a totally natural one, there must be *someone* to blame—someone who had committed either errors of commission or errors of omission. The medicolegal net was so finely and densely woven that normal everyday discussion of bad news appeared almost impossible.

The situation has improved greatly over the last decade or so; nevertheless, there is still a fear of medicolegal consequences hanging over any discussion of bad news, and the feeling of "I'd like to tell this patient the facts about the medical condition, but will I be held responsible if I do?"

Furthermore, the ambiguity of the word *sorry* has added to the difficulty. The word *sorry* has two distinct meanings. When one says, "I am sorry for you," it is an expression of the feeling that is commonly termed *sympathy,* but when one says, "I am sorry that I did this," it implies regret and in turn responsibility (or in medicolegal terms *culpability* or *exposure*). Hence, even when we begin to express human sympathy for the feelings of the other person, we may inadvertently be accepting responsibility if we say, "I am sorry," instead of the clearer but clumsier "I am sorry for the way you're feeling."

Another advantage of the empathic response—as you will see shortly—is that it makes explicit the emotion that is being expressed and the immediate cause of that emotion. By stating overtly the connection between the two, a sentence such as "This is clearly awful for you" avoids the ambiguities entailed in the simple single word *sorry.*

6. DEALING WITH HOPE

It is often stated as a maxim of medical practice that we should "never take away all hope." Professionals who find these conversations difficult have often used this principle as a reason (or, more accurately, an excuse) for not telling the truth to patients or for avoiding serious discussion about adverse events. The rationalization is that by telling the patient nothing, you are protecting him or her from losing all hope in the aftermath of the news.

Now, this difficulty—the fear of destroying hope—is at its greatest if we erroneously equate truth telling with the destruction of all hope. If you happen to think that disclosure of a diagnosis that includes the word *cancer,* for example, is tantamount to abolishing all hope, then you will avoid using the word (as more than 90 percent of physicians did in the 1960s).[2]

In practice, discussing the facts by no means necessarily implies the abolition of all hope. The central purpose of the SPIKES protocol is to enable you to discuss the medical facts openly and honestly and at the same time acknowledge the impact that those facts produce. This process could be termed *sensitive truth telling* and contrasts starkly with the older ways of dealing with bad news. Even as late as the 1970s, doctors either concealed information (perhaps best described as *sensitive concealment* or *protective patronizing*) or, more rarely, blurted out the bad news, which could perhaps be termed *insensitive truth telling* (i.e., stating the facts without regard to their impact on the patient).

We can legitimately claim to have made considerable progress in clinical communication since then. Any way you look at it, however, dealing with hope is never easy. As we shall see later, the important point to remember is that hope is not a single monolithic entity. There are many components that make up any individual's hope in a situation, some of which may be unobtainable (as, for example, cure may be), while other hopes are realistic and are directed at goals that can be reached (for example, control of many physical symptoms, fixing the fear of being abandoned, and resolving family conflicts, to name a few).

The problem of dealing with hope is not trivial, and you will find a longer discussion of this topic in section 2.5. We need to be aware of the fear of abolishing all hope as a mental deterrent to our breaking bad news.

7. CHALLENGES TO DEATH DENIAL

It has been suggested that, for many of us, part of the reason we decided on a career in health care was to diminish our own personal anxieties about disease and death. Of course, the importance of this particular motive in our own psychological makeup varies enormously: for some of us, the motive of death denial is important, while for others it may not play a material role at all. Whether this motive plays a big or a small role, a discussion about disease progression or terminal illness will challenge any denial that we may have about death. Further, the more that we seem to have in common with the patient, the greater this challenge is. If the patient reminds you strongly of yourself, it becomes even more difficult to avoid the hidden implied threat to your own view of your future ("There, but for fortune . . ." or "the grace of God . . .").

Hence, identifying with the plight of the patient, which in itself has many potential benefits for both parties, also carries with it the potential hazard of challenging our own view of our future. Simply being aware of this factor is helpful, and may partly negate its effect as an obstacle in breaking bad news.

8. LOCAL CONFLICTS

On top of all that, there are problems created by what we might call "local medical politics," in other words, the local influences of other people that may conflict over the patient and his/her clinical care.

For example, you may not be aware of the views expressed, or of implicit promises made, by other physicians involved in the patient's care. There is a fuller discussion of this in section 6.2. ("But the surgeon said he got it all.")

Sometimes, of course, the local turbulence arises not from other professionals but from the patient's family members. Again, there is fuller discussion of this topic in section 6.2. ("My mother is not to be told.")

Curiously enough, there are answers to some of the fundamental questions about sharing information. To put it simply, we are all obliged to tell any patient who is mentally competent, orientated, and above the age of consent any information about his or her condition that the patient asks for. In other words, if a patient asks, we are obliged to tell.

However, we are not obliged to give details, including the diagnosis, if the patient specifically does not want the information given to her or him. However, most ethicists would agree that even if a mentally competent patient does not want the diagnosis named, we are obliged to describe the seriousness of the condition, the nature of the treatment we propose and the consequences of not getting that treatment, as well as the consequences (including side effects) of receiving the treatment.

Most authorities would agree that those are our obligations. Of course, other circumstances have an influence: for example, most clinical trials specify in the entry criteria that the patient must know the diagnosis (particularly true in oncology). If the patient does not want the diagnosis named or discussed, entry to that clinical trial is not possible, although, of course, treatment for that condition is possible with regimens outside the clinical trial.

Furthermore, most authorities would agree that if a patient insists on not knowing the diagnosis—a rare event nowadays, but it still happens occasionally—we are obliged to ask if there is someone else (a daughter or son or a close friend, perhaps) with whom the patient would like us to discuss the diagnosis or treatment. In many cases, but not in all, there is another person with whom we will be asked to talk. Even so, a few times in my career I have looked after patients who specified that they did not want the diagnosis named and were comfortable making decisions about the treatment and other aspects of care without any third party being involved.

As we shall see in chapter 3, there is only one choice when it comes to disclosing medical errors. In that situation there is an obligation— moral, ethical, and in many places, legal—to disclose any significant error, whether serious harm has occurred or not.

As you will see in the next section, the SPIKES protocol includes an invitation to share the information, so that if the patient specifically does not want the information at that moment, you can leave it with them. In chapter 3, I describe the CONES protocol for error disclosure for use when there is an obligation to describe the situation.

2.3. The SPIKES Protocol: "Before You Tell, Ask"

The heart of the six-step SPIKES protocol lies in the idea that the P—for hearing the patient's Perception—comes before the K (for knowledge, i.e., the medical facts).

This section explains each of the six main steps. After that I suggest a few specific strategies that may help when discussing the prognosis in particular settings.

S: Setting and Starting

To start the interview off well, it works in your favor if you can arrange the physical setting—the physical surroundings or context—of the interview to make the surroundings as conducive as possible to a helpful discussion.

It may seem fussy, but a few seconds spent on these factors make a great deal of difference. They help, first of all, because they help you. Because you are exercising control over some of the aspects of the interview, you are going to feel a bit more confident and comfortable. They also help the patient because when you look a bit more comfortable, confident, and in control, that equates in the patient's mind with increased competence.

For that reason, it's worth making a little extra effort to start the interaction off well. I discussed that in greater detail in table 1.1, but I will repeat the information in table 2.1 so that you don't have to flip back and forth.

P: Perception

Having optimized the setting (the physical components) of the interaction, you then need to find out what the patient understands—or suspects—of her or his situation. In other words, you need to hear from the patient what she or he has been told or suspects and/or thinks of the current situation. Clearly, there is a difference between patients who are new to you and patients whom you know (and who may be, for example, coming back to hear the results of tests that you have ordered).

For that reason, I shall split this section on *P* for *Perception* into two parts: the first for when you are talking with patients who are new to you, and the second for when you talking with patients whom you already know.

When the Patient and/or Clinical Situation Is New to You

The objective is relatively straightforward—to find out what the patient knows, suspects, or thinks. The actual words that you use in assessing the patient's perception are not crucial. There is no "magic formula" of words that suits every person or works every time. Here are a few easy examples of phrases you can use. The idea behind all of them is the same, and you can use these or any phrasing that feels comfortable to you:

Examples of Assessing Perception with a New Patient
- "So what do you make of the situation?"
- "What did Dr. X tell you when he/she sent you here?"

TABLE 2.1   *A Few Basic Tips*

Technique	Central Feature	Notes
Greeting	Use the person's name.	A simple way of establishing the "person" as well as the "problem"
Introduce yourself	Briefly say who you are and what you do.	Merely courteous
Shake hands	Make actual contact.	Don't do that if you have a cold.
Sit down!	Bring your eyes to the same level as the other person's.	Essential
Don't be too far away	Have less than four feet of space between you.	The optimal distance varies with gender and culture, but three feet is rarely wrong.
Adopt a neutral body posture	Look relaxed, or at least not too anxious or irritated.	Even if you don't feel relaxed (and most of us don't at these times), try to adopt the neutral body posture and look relaxed.
Lean forward	Don't sit back all the way against the chair.	Studies show that patients recognize this as a sign of being interested in them.
Be ready to smile	Smiling may not be your usual "thing," but it helps if you can manage it.	If you do smile, try to "smile with your whole face."
Switch on your listening skills	Silence and repetition	Consciously maintain silence as the patient starts talking. Then in your first sentence of response use a word or phrase from the patient's last sentence.

- "When you first had that chest pain/found that breast lump, did you think it was something serious?"
- "Why don't you tell me what you understand about the situation, and I'll go on from there."
- "Tell me what you think is going on."
- "What have you been told about the medical situation?"
- "Tell me what you've been thinking about the medical situation."

As the patient replies and describes what he or she knows or has been told, there are two important things for you to listen for:

1. THE VOCABULARY AND THE COMPREHENSION

Try to assess at what level the patient understands the situation. Nowadays, many patients might say something like, "They said it was breast cancer, less than two centimeters, and it hadn't spread to the lymph nodes, and it did have those hormone receptors on it." It is valuable to hear this from the patient because so much of the work has already been done for you, and you can start with, "That's right. Now, if it's less than two centimeters we'd regard that as quite small, which is good, and when it hasn't spread to the lymph nodes, that's also good."

On the other hand, occasionally a patient with, for example, lung cancer will say something like, "My primary care doctor said they saw some nodes on the chest x-ray, but it didn't sound serious or anything." In that case, you clearly have a lot of work to do because the gap between perception and reality is wide.

As the patient describes his or her level of comprehension, make a quick mental note of the type of words the person uses so that you can later align your description of the situation (discussed in the section on *K* for *K*nowledge) with the patient's perception. So, if he or she uses the phrase "little bits of calcium," you can start by explaining that "little bits of calcium" might indicate something serious or might not. This process of aligning your language is a good way of responding to the patient, and it is helpful in building the relationship between the two of you.

2. THE PRESENCE OF DENIAL

It sometimes—but rarely—happens that the patient says that he or she has not been told anything when the referring physician has told you otherwise. Clearly, the patient is exhibiting denial, and when this happens (even though you might be holding the referring letter stating that the diagnosis has been discussed), you simply need to note the denial, just as you would note any other symptom such as pain. You need not (and should not) confront the denial directly at this stage. So, if the patient says, "They didn't tell me anything at that other clinic," it would not be a good idea to reply, "Oh, yes, they did! They told you your lungs were wearing out, and even *then* you wouldn't give up smoking." It is much more helpful to acknowledge the patient's perception of what he or she was told (i.e., that the patient believes that he or she was told nothing) and then go on to ask the patient (in the *I-In*vitation step; see below) what he or she would like to know about the condition now.

When the Patient Is Known to You

When the patient is known to you—if, for example, the patient is returning to see you to hear the results of tests that have been done—this part of the interview can be much briefer. In fact, I suggest that you can simply and quickly check on the patient's perception and elicit an invitation to go on and share information, in one relatively brief and simple response.

Even though such a response is brief, it is worth doing in all situations in which the news is bad. I deal with this combination (of *P* for *Perception* and *I* for *Invitation*) in patients who are known to you in the latter part of the next section (after I have talked about eliciting an invitation in patients who are new to you).

I: Invitation

The invitation to share the information may be brief, but it is nevertheless important. The objective of this part of the interview is to get agreement from the patient for you to share the information, the bad news.

Because the emphasis is slightly different when the patient is new to you than it is when a patient is known, I deal with these two types of situation separately.

When the Patient and/or Clinical Situation Is New to You

At the moment when you offer the patient medical facts, you are, of course, simultaneously offering the patient a chance *not* to hear the exact details of the diagnosis if that is what he or she wishes. (See chapter 3 for examples of the opposite—situations in which you have to tell.) Even if the invitation is as slight as, "I'd like to tell you the results of the test. Is that OK?" you are still involving the patient in taking the next step. You are performing shared decision making.

The exact words you use are not critical, and I have set out a few examples below. What is important is that for those few seconds you are asking for the patient's collaboration. It may sound like a simple matter or courtesy or even common sense, but it will not be forgotten.

Examples of Eliciting an Invitation When the Patient Is New to You
- "How would you like me to deal with this?"
- "Shall I tell you what we know so far?"
- "Is it OK if I go ahead and tell you what we know about your situation so far?"
- "Are you the kind of person who'd like to know the details as far as we know them?"
- "I'll go ahead and talk about the results of the biopsy/ECG/scan. Is that OK?"
- "How would you like me to handle the information? Shall I go ahead and tell you what we know?"

When the Patient and Clinical Situation Are Known to You
The difference in breaking bad news when you know the patient and her or his situation is, of course, the shared history of your contacts.

With a new patient, you do not have a shared history; with a patient who is known to you, you do. In other words, when the patient is new to you, as we have just seen, it is important to find out what the person knows or suspects about the condition before you tell the diagnosis. In that situation, with the new patient, you are starting "from scratch."

But when the patient is in follow-up, it is still helpful to do a similar thing, although you can do it more briefly. You can achieve this by giving a short précis—a "recap"—of the situation and immediately going on to set the agenda for sharing information. For example, you can give a one-phrase summary of why you ordered the test (or whatever), before going straight on to check that it's all right with the person if you discuss the findings. (See below.)

As you give the recap of the situation, you can check with the patient that this accords with his or her understanding. In other words, you can make sure that you are both "on the same page" and then go on to say that you are going to discuss the results.

Now, this may not seem like a big matter, but it makes a big difference to the interview. In giving that quick recap of the shared background, you are doing two valuable things. First, you are reminding this particular patient that you are aware of your shared history—that you have not forgotten the patient or his or her story. Second, you are taking control of the interview. You are obeying the motto "Act, don't react"; you are taking your own action rather than making a reflex reaction. In doing that, you are putting yourself in a better position to offer support (including the use of empathic responses) in what follows, as we shall see.

Following that, the invitation to share the information can be brief—almost rhetorical. In fact, it is usually more a matter of setting the agenda ("I'll go ahead and tell you what the scan showed. Is that OK?") rather than a full and more formal invitation. Even though it is brief, however, it is still valuable and shows the patient that he or she does have a role in the process. The decision making is shared, in the sense that the patient could (in theory) back out of the process and stop you from delivering the news.

Here are a few examples of how you can clarify the patient's perception and then go on to set the agenda:

Examples of Clarifying Perception and Then Invitation to Discuss Results with a Patient in Follow-up
- "Remember that because of that pain in your abdomen I was concerned that something might be going on in the liver? And I thought a CT would help. So I'll tell you what it shows, OK?"
- "That back pain didn't seem to have an obvious explanation, and I thought the bone scan might help us. Shall I go ahead and tell you what it shows?"
- "Just to go over why I wanted the blood tests: remember, I was wondering if there was some reason for your high blood pressure, so we did the tests. Shall I tell you all the results now?"
- "To recap why I wanted the CT scan: When the urine tests showed blood repeatedly, I wanted the CT to see if there was anything going on in the bladder or the kidneys. So I'll go over the results with you, OK?"

As you can see from those examples, when you know the patient, the recap can be brief, and then you may need to ask for only a brief confirmation of the agenda you propose. Even so, as I have said, this is a valuable thing to do.

To sum up, then, there is only a small difference between the way you ask when you know the patient and the way you ask when the patient is new. Although the difference is small and is a matter of emphasis rather than a different task, it is nonetheless worth doing. Some form of invitation or agenda setting does help before you go ahead with the information sharing. (An analogy I often use is to consider the way a man might phrase a marriage proposal. There is a big difference between "Will you marry me on Saturday?" and "We're getting married on Saturday.")

The few seconds that you spend on a recap of past events and on agenda setting will make it much easier for the patient to cope with the information. It is a good investment of your time.

What If the Patient Asks Immediately?

It happens often that the patient will jump in with an anxious question about the test results even before you have sat down. You should acknowledge the anxiety immediately (with an empathic response; see below) and then go on to the "*P and I*" combination.

Let's say you ordered a CT scan to investigate abdominal pain and on the return visit the patient asks, "What did the CT scan show?" You will find it more helpful to respond by acknowledging the anxiety and going straight on to a recap with something such as, "I realize this is a big worry, and I'm going to tell you the results. Remember when you had that pain in your abdomen I was concerned that something might be going on the liver?" (A few other examples follow below.)

Saying something like that takes a short time, but it reminds the patient of the reason for the test, and it also allows you to set the agenda for the next few minutes, thus taking control of the interview. This in turn allows you to be more supportive and helpful to the patient's response to the news when you come to it.

Examples of Responding to an Immediate and Anxious Question about Test Results
- "I realize that that's important. Remember we did the CT to see what was going on? Well, let me tell you what it shows, OK?"
- "This is important, and I'll tell you. Remember we were focusing on the liver to see if there was an explanation for the pain you had? I'll tell you what it shows, OK?"
- "I know that's a big issue and has obviously been worrying you. Let me tell you what the CT showed, OK? Remember we were

trying to find out if anything was going on in the liver? Well, the CT shows . . ."

- "Obviously very important. And I realize you've been worried. We did the CT to try to find out what was causing the pain in your abdomen. I'll tell you the results, OK?"

Saying something like that takes a short time, but it reminds the patient of the reason for the test, and—a factor that is just as important—it allows you to set the agenda for the next few minutes, thus taking control of the interview. This in turn allows you to be more supportive and helpful to the patient's response to the news when you come to it.

K: Knowledge

Having obtained a clear invitation to share the information—or at least agreement to the agenda that you have proposed—you can now start giving the medical facts. As you do so, there are a few rules or guidelines that may help you. (See table 2.2.)

Align Your Language with the Patient's Vocabulary

As you begin to describe the bad news, try to use the same type of vocabulary that you hear the patient use in describing his or her perception of the situation. So, if the patient says "a shadow," you can start with the

TABLE 2.2   *Some Guidelines for Giving Information*

Align your language with the patient's vocabulary.	Use similar (or the same) words at the same level as you've heard the patient use.
Give the information in small chunks.	Don't give a long monologue. The patient may "drift off" or be totally at sea.
Check the patient's understanding.	You can use questions such as "Does that make sense?" "Do you follow me?" "Is that clear so far?".
Use plain language, not technical jargon.	It is an effort to deliberately translate technical "Medspeak" into everyday language, but it is worthwhile.
Respond to the patient's intense emotions as they are expressed.	See next section E—Emotions.

word *shadow* and say something like, "Yes, and I don't know if it was mentioned, but shadows can be caused by several different things, some serious, some not." Or if the patient says, "Apparently, it's type 2 diabetes, and my BMI is 35, which is a problem," you can start there: "That's right. And that body mass index—as I'm sure they said—means that we *really* have to get your weight down, which might get the diabetes to go away completely."

Some examples (of the many hundreds of words in Medspeak that need translation) are included in table 2.3. Obviously, you don't have to use these types of words if the patient clearly understands what you are saying, but sometimes when you're searching for a plain language version, words and phrases like these may be useful.

Give the Information in Small Chunks
This is an important guideline for giving information: *Give the facts in small chunks.* Try to avoid a long monologue (even though you might be justifiably proud of the amount you know about the condition). Try consciously to stop every few sentences and check that the patient is still with you and "on the same page."

One major reason for doing this is because if you do not, the patient may "drift away" and start thinking about the worst possible consequences of your opening statement. While you are trying at length to present the rather reassuring facts about, let's say, ductal cancer in situ of the breast, the patient might well be imagining the worst possible consequences associated with the word *cancer*. That's why it is so useful to stop yourself giving a long monologue by checking that the patient understands what you are saying.

Check the Patient's Understanding
The words that you use to make sure your patient is getting the message are entirely a matter of your own style. Here are a few examples, some of which I use frequently and many of which my colleagues also use often.

Examples of Checking the Patient's Understanding
- "Do you follow me?"
- "Is this all making sense so far?"

TABLE 2.3   *Translating Medspeak into Plain Language*

Medspeak	Plain Language
Negative	Doesn't show anything wrong
Progression	Getting worse
Morphologically	Under the microscope
Metastatic screen	Tests done to see if there has been any spread
Performance	How much you can do (for example, how many flights of stairs)
Equivocal	Can't be certain what it means
Lung consolidation	Pneumonia
Compliance	Get through the treatment
Upper respiratory tract infection	Cold (or sore throat)
Ecchymosis	Bruise
Postural drop	Blood pressure goes down when you stand up
Imaging	X-ray or CT scan (or whatever it is)
Partial remission	Getting smaller
Undifferentiated	More aggressive than the average
Fibrosis	Scar tissue
Neutropenia	Low white-cell count
Nephropathy	Affecting the kidneys
Lesion	Something wrong
Titrating	Adjusting the dose
Purpura	Pinpoints of bleeding
Vasovagal	Usual type of faint
The bone scan is negative.	The bone scan doesn't show anything wrong.
There is renal dysfunction.	Your kidneys are not working normally.
The metastatic potential	The chance of its spreading
Hypertension	High blood pressure
Hematuria	Blood in your urine
Ascites	Fluid in your abdomen
There are multiple opacities on the CT.	There are a lot of shadows on the CT.
Equivocal significance	We don't know if it matters or not.
Ischemic heart disease	Problems with your coronary arteries
It is lymph node positive.	It has spread to the lymph nodes.

- "Does that make sense?"
- "OK?"
- "Do you see what I mean?"
- "Any questions so far?"
- "OK so far?"
- "Do you get the general picture?"

Use Plain Language, Not Technical Jargon

Of all the guidelines about sharing information, perhaps the one that requires the greatest effort is making sure that you express the facts in plain language, not in esoteric technical jargon. The basic problem is that our medical technical jargon is useful for rapid transmission of information, but it is usually unintelligible to the patient. For example, in a medical emergency, our technical jargon—sometimes called Medspeak—is a brilliant and efficient way of transferring a large amount of information in a few words. Think of how much information is carried in "Chemotherapy ten days ago. WBC now 0.2. Temp is 39.2. The systolic is 80 and falling." In a few seconds, you have an accurate picture of probable septic shock.

We are justifiably proud of our ability to speak and understand Medspeak; it is unambiguous, precise, hard to learn (at first), and immensely valuable. The problem is that our patients don't speak it or understand it, so we must make a conscious effort to translate what we want to say into plain language.

Of course, some patients will want to move the vocabulary up to the technical level. For that reason, you can, if you wish, use the technical word first and then translate it into plain language. For example, you might say, "The bone scan is reported as negative. That means it doesn't show anything wrong." This shows that you clearly know the technical words, but you are also making an effort to ensure the patient understands the meaning. Table 2.4 translates some technical ideas into plain language.

TABLE 2.4 *Translating Technical Ideas into Plain Language*

The Technical Idea	Examples of Useful Phrases
Clinical trial	Comparison of a new treatment with the standard one that everyone uses at the moment
Randomization	The electronic equivalent of flipping a coin so there's no bias as to who gets which treatment
Axillary node sampling	Taking some lymph nodes from the armpit to see if there has been any spread
Sentinel node biopsy	Taking just a few of the nodes nearest the breast
Neoadjuvant therapy	Treatment given before the surgery to try to shrink the tumor

This is why it is so valuable to check that your patient understands what you are saying (using phrases that are on the same lines as the ones in the Check Understanding section above). If you check with the patient and the patient does understand and is comfortable with the technical words, it is relatively simple to shift up from plain language to technical language thereafter. On the other hand, if you don't check with the patient, it is difficult to shift down (from technical jargon to plain language) because you will not necessarily know that the patient doesn't get it.

E: Emotions

As has been mentioned many times already, responding to the emotional content of the interaction is the key to a supportive doctor-patient relationship. If the patient experiences a strong emotion and the doctor does not seem to notice, the patient will regard the doctor as cold or insensitive. That rule applies to every stage of the interview, right from the start, particularly if (as we have already seen) the patient asks an anxious question as he or she enters the room.

The point of this technique is that the simple process of *acknowledging the emotion* often is all that is needed in emotion handling. In everyday practice, *responding to the emotion often means no more than acknowledging it,* telling the patient that you have noticed the emotion and its cause. The easiest and more straightforward way of doing this is the empathic response (as discussed in section 1.2). To make life easier, I set out the same text here to save your having to flip back and forth.

STEP 1: IDENTIFY ONE OF THE EMOTIONS
Most of us experience a mixture of several emotions at the same time. For example, on hearing a piece of bad news, we may feel some fear, some anger, and some disappointment, and we might also have difficulty comprehending it (disbelief) or even want to shut out the news (denial). All of those emotions might coexist behind a shocked "Oh, no!"

So when the patient shows an emotional response (such as "Oh, no!"), you simply need to decide on *one* of the emotions that you can see. (And the fact that you can see the emotional expression clearly shows that it is a "big" experience, something the patient feels intensely and deeply.)

Having fixed on one of the emotions in the mixture, name it (in your own mind). Say to yourself, "This patient is clearly shocked," or "He's angry now," or "She's having difficulty believing what I just said." Don't be afraid of using words with wide, all-inclusive meanings, such as *shock* or *distress* or *upset* and so on.

STEP 2: IDENTIFY THE CAUSE OF THE EMOTION

Usually the cause of the emotion is the piece of news that you have just given or the topic that one of you has just raised. That is all you need. You don't need to perform some miracle of psychoanalysis ("This man is upset because he now sees his career and relationships as total failures and is doubtful that he can recreate his lost youth"). All you need do in step 2 is to pinpoint the immediate cause of the emotional reaction; often it will be something that you have just said.

STEP 3: RESPOND IN A WAY THAT SHOWS YOU HAVE MADE THE CONNECTION BETWEEN STEPS 1 AND 2

Tell the patient that you have observed his or her feelings and that you are aware of what evoked that emotion. Empathic responses (and there are hundreds, of course!) are usually in the form of "Clearly, that's a major shock," or "You are obviously upset by this," or "I realize that this is awful for you," or "This is difficult to take in, isn't it?"

When you respond to a patient's feelings with an empathic response, you achieve three objectives simultaneously:

1. *You legitimize that person's feelings.* You are telling the patient that the emotion he or she is experiencing *is* an understandable response to the situation. In doing that, you are showing that you not making a judgment about the emotion.

2. *You are telling the person that it is permissible to discuss those feelings.* You are demonstrating that feelings are legitimate items on the agenda between the two of you. In the words of the cliché: "We can talk about this."

3. *You change the subject.* For that moment, you are not talking about the infarct or the hypertension or the bowel cancer; you are talking about how the person *feels* at this moment in response to that information.

In other words, you are showing the patient that you have noted his or her feelings, however briefly, and are including those emotions as part of your overall approach to the clinical situation.

The empathic response, by simply identifying the emotion that is there, is nonjudgmental. You may (appropriately) be forming a judgment of the situation in your own mind (you may be thinking, "This patient is making a big fuss over a small problem"), but your response does not express the judgment. When you make an empathic response, you are not stating that judgment of the emotion and you not stating whether the emotion is appropriate (in your view) or in proportion (in your view) to the import of the news. You are simply stating that you have seen that the patient is experiencing it. That's one of the main features of the empathic response—you are acknowledging the existence of the patient's emotion and not stating your own assessment of the appropriateness of that emotion.

Here is an example (from another physician's recent practice) in which the escalation response clearly is judgmental and (as actually happened) led to the patient's strong feeling that the doctor was not helpful or supportive.

➤ *Situation:*
The patient has small-cell lung cancer, presenting at an advanced stage. You explain that it can be controlled for a time, but cannot be cured.

The Patient Says:
"Oh, my god! You mean you can't fix it? You can't cure it?"
You Can Choose From:
—*Direct or Factual Response*
   "That's right; sadly, there are virtually no cures."
—*Escalationary or Judgmental Response*
   "You're not coping with this very well, are you?"
—*Open Question*
   "What's going through your mind at the moment?"
—*Empathic Response*
   "This is clearly a big shock, isn't it?"

To make that point again: the empathic response is valuable as the first response to an immediate reaction. It may well have been that (as in this example) the patient was not coping well with the news. Even so, making a statement of that assessment as the first response to the patient's reaction did in fact lead to a marked deterioration in the relationship with the doctor and made later management much more difficult than necessary. In the next example, I compare the empathic response to other ways of responding to an immediate and anxious question about a bone scan that was done because of low back pain.

➤ *Situation:*
The patient had a mastectomy for breast cancer four years ago and has now had two weeks of back pain with no precipitating cause. You have done a bone scan, which, unfortunately, shows multiple bone metastases.

> *The Patient Says:*
> "What did the bone scan show?" (She says this immediately and anxiously as you enter the room.)
> *You Can Choose From:*
> —*Direct or Factual Response*
>   "I'm afraid it shows that the cancer has come back."
> —*Escalationary or Judgmental Response*
>   "Don't rush me. I'll get to it in a minute."
> —*Open Question*
>   "Tell me what you have been thinking is going on?"
> —*Empathic Response*
>   "I know you're worried, and I'll tell you what it showed. You remember I ordered the bone scan to find out if there had been any recurrence . . ."

It is worth noting that there is nothing intrinsically (or even morally) wrong or ill advised about answering with the direct/factual response, but, depending on the emotional state of the patient, it might be followed by a strong emotional reaction for which neither of you has prepared. By acknowledging the initial emotion (anxiety) and then proceeding for a few seconds with a brief assessment of perception and then setting the agenda, you take control of the interview, and you and the patient are both a little more ready to deal with the emotion. In the words of a common maxim, you "act rather than react."

S: Strategy and Summary

Perhaps the most important feature of the SPIKES protocol is that the second S, for Strategy and Summary, comes *after* the E for Emotion. If the patient is experiencing a strong emotion, he or she will not be able to listen to or focus on your proposed plan of management until after the emotion has been acknowledged. Until you have acknowledged the presence of the strong emotion—the elephant in the room, as it were—the patient will not be able to focus on what you are saying about the management plan. An unacknowledged strong emotion produces a paralyzing effect until the emotion has been acknowledged. That is why *S* for *Strategy and Summary* comes *after* the E for acknowledging Emotion—and not instead of it.

Explaining the Clinical Strategy

The secret of a workable clinical strategy or management plan is to try as well as you can to have the patient "buy into" it. The best way of doing that is to attempt to match, as far as is possible, what you propose to do with the patient's greatest concerns. For example, if you are starting treatment with antihypertensive medications and the patient has already indicated that he is worried about possible side effects, you can acknowledge that as you explain the strategy. You might say something such as, "I know you're worried about side effects, so what I suggest is we start with this medication, and if you have problems with it, we'll change to another one after, say, two weeks. Does that make sense?"

Summarizing at the End of the Interview

It is important to end the interview properly. In the retail trades, this is called "closure of sale." Most business people are taught about it and are far better at this part than we are in clinical medicine. In fact, the closing of the interview is not as difficult as you might fear.

There are three main components of an effective closing:

1. A summary in a couple of sentences of what has been discussed.
2. "Any questions for right now?"
3. An arrangement for the next meeting ("a contract for the next contact").

Summarizing ten minutes of conversation in a few sentences requires some thought! As the French philosopher Pascal said in one of his letters, "I'm sorry this is such a long letter. I haven't got the time to write a short one." His point was a good one; making a brief précis of what you have discussed in the previous minutes does require a bit of mental effort. But it gets easier with practice. The more often that you do it, the easier and more natural it becomes. You might say something like, "So, the tests show that there is no particular reason for having high blood pressure. We'll start the treatment with this tablet and then you let me know if you have any problems or side effects with it."

Almost always in discussing bad news, the patient has some questions or concerns at the back of his or her mind, and you should ask about them even if you have no time to answer fully right now. You can easily note the issues and say something like, "That's obviously important—we must talk about that in detail next time." This is, after all, how psychiatrists handle what they called the "fifty-ninth minute issue"—the question that is raised by the patient right at the end of the hour-long session (probably for subconscious reasons). The psychiatrist simply tells the patient that the issue should be the top item on the agenda for next time. You can use the same technique, unless, of course, the issue that the patient mentions is potentially major. ("Oh, by the way, I've been coughing up blood for a week.")

Patients almost always feel that the interview is incomplete if there are issues that have not even been raised. By setting the agenda for next time, you have also reinforced the fact that there will be a next time, which reinforces the continuing relationship between the two of you.

Close the interview with a clear arrangement for the next meeting (if there is one). This need not be protracted or fancy; it can be as simple as "So I'll see you in two weeks." It is a simple and straightforward contract for the next contact. Then, as you part, it is a matter of simple courtesy to say "Goodbye" or "Goodbye for now" or "See you next time."

Those, then, are the six main steps of the SPIKES strategy for breaking bad news. Now let's look at a few of the commonest types of reactions that patients and relatives express, and consider how you might respond to them.

2.4. Some Reactions to Bad News

Is the Patient's Response Adaptive or Maladaptive?

As the patient responds to the bad news, the main feature of the response that we need to focus on is whether it is making the situation better or worse. This is the criterion behind the idea of regarding a response as either adaptive or maladaptive.

To put it simply, an adaptive response is one that reduces the stress or the impact of the situation. In other words, it is a coping strategy.

As I shall discuss, some responses that are unhelpful in the long term—such as denial—may be of help to the patient in the short term. Temporary denial may be a way of postponing the action of handling bad news that seems initially to be overwhelming and devastating.

In a similar way, many responses that we all encounter in clinical practice contain some elements that are adaptive and other elements that are maladaptive.

Some Responses That Are Usually Adaptive (Helpful)

Organizing and planning. Making pragmatic plans for the immediate future is always adaptive. The process of planning and prioritizing actions restores a sense of perspective.

Hope. Realistic hope usually helps the patient cope and is regarded as adaptive. However, prolonged *unrealistic* hope may be maladaptive.

Humor. Some people—but not all—habitually use humor to help them cope with threats. Provided it comes after taking in the medical facts (and not instead of doing that), it is usually adaptive and reduces stress.

Some Responses That Are Usually Maladaptive (Unhelpful)

Despair. Despair is a word derived from Latin and means "loss of hope" (i.e., hopelessness). As such, it is an emotion triggered by a cognitive act—the act of understanding the medical fact. The emotion of despair is an unpleasant one and in itself is a condition or a secondary diagnosis precipitated by the medical condition.

Guilt. It often seems to me that if the world could magically and totally obliterate just one emotion, the best candidate for annihilation would be guilt (closely followed by despair). I regard guilt as a common but always maladaptive feeling that adds to the burden of the medical situation and never provides benefit.

Prolonged denial. Some people (myself included) regard *short-lived* denial as one type of normal response to a threatening condition. If you see it that way, then you will not regard a short period of denial as maladaptive or pathological but will regard *prolonged denial* as maladaptive in the sense that the patient is not coping in a helpful manner with—and so not adapting to—the new circumstances.

Prolonged hope. As with denial, so with hope. Prolonged unrealistic hope can lead to inappropriate decisions and plans and can legitimately be regarded as maladaptive.

Anxiety-provoking quest. Often, as I shall discuss further in the section on displacement behavior, taking on a quest can be a mechanism that helps the patient focus and organize. Sometimes, however, the quest is simply too big and far reaching, and it may then induce performance anxiety and distress in the patient who now feels that he or she is not measuring up to the stated goals. In that sense, therefore, a quest can sometimes be simply "too much" and might produce a sense of despair and might legitimately be regarded as maladaptive.

Some Responses That Are Neither Adaptive nor Maladaptive

Fear. The function of fear as an intellectual activity is rarely discussed. Of course, the adrenergic fight-or-flight reaction is of great value to the individual faced with a physical danger. The problem is that the release of those hormones also triggers an intellectual and emotional reaction that we call fear (the intellectual correlate of stress). I do not regard fear as either adaptive or maladaptive in itself. I regard ordinary fear (as opposed to an anxiety attack) as a common emotion triggered by an intellectual perception of something perceived as a threat—and hence the emotional part of the intellectual activity of taking in the adverse news.

Perhaps we can look more closely at that by using an example of the situation in which you have had to tell the patient that there is a strong possibility of their dying. In that situation, which naturally precipitates fear in the great majority of patients, a very small number of people are so well adjusted to the prospect of dying that they genuinely have no fear. I have met perhaps three such patients in my entire career. In the rest of such cases, one's first thought on encountering a patient who seems to have no fear should be, "Does this patient understand the implications of this news?" I discuss methods of dealing with the expressions of fear in the section on it below.

Psychological Shock. As distinct from the hemodynamic meaning of the same word, psychological shock is the psychological equivalent of a bruise. Just as a bruise can be caused by a fall, a blunt object, a blow, or a sprain, so shock can be caused by many different types of events. Shock can be the end result of a surge of fear, anger, disappointment, or loss, among other feelings. It is a sign of damage or impact and is commensurate with the force of the psychological impact and with the sensitivity of the normal processes (the equivalent of the tissues in a bruise) to trauma. In the same way as some people bruise more easily than others, some experience shock more easily and with less provocation than others. Like a bruise, shock will often fade over time.

Disbelief. Disbelief is also a reaction that can legitimately be regarded as "within the normal range." Perhaps the word *disbelief* implies that the patient is having *difficulty* taking the information on board although she or he consciously wants to. Seen in this way, we can regard disbelief as a common and normal response to bad news, and it is a response that needs to be noted and acknowledged (some examples follow).

Denial. The word *denial* implies that the person is not able to take in the information and that the inability is often unconscious (as opposed to *disbelief,* when the person is aware of the difficulty in accepting the facts). Perhaps we could say that disbelief is comparable to "I can't, even though I'm trying," while denial is comparable to "I won't, and I may not even be aware of my block."

In either event—whether the individual's response is better classified as disbelief or denial—the important thing to note is that both of these responses are normal *in the short term.* It is when disbelief or denial is *prolonged* over a period of time, and discussions about the situation are not possible because of the patient's state, that problems arise.

Displacement and "the quest." A displacement activity is an activity that the patient undertakes instead of coping with the problem. The signal features are that displacement activities take a considerable amount of time and effort. Similarly, some people set themselves a major quest—picking a monumental task that is going to require a major amount of effort in the future.

In many ways, displacement activities—doing things that are not immediately relevant to the news—are common and not abnormal. Many patients focus in the short term on an activity that is not necessarily relevant to their own situation. Most often this decreases the sense of distress and can thus be regarded as adaptive. Only when the displacement activity or a major quest causes new and additional distress should it be regarded as maladaptive.

What Matters to the Patient

What matters to the patient is whether or not this particular response is *helping him or her* at this particular time.

In many respects, it doesn't matter so much what *we* think of our patient's reactions—whether or not we consider them appropriate or inappropriate—what matters is the effect of this particular reaction on the situation.

This way of looking at things is, in itself, important and will probably change your behavior. It is useful to stop measuring the patient's responses by some preordained standard (in other words, to avoid being judgmental) but instead to examine whether the reaction is making things worse or better for this particular patient. This in turn will help you make an empathic response—acknowledging the emotion and what the patient is going through—instead of deciding whether or not it is appropriate. In the "crossroads" examples below, the response labeled as Escalation Response is usually prompted by a prejudgment of what is appropriate and therefore expected (see also the "crossroads" example above: "You're not coping very well, are you?").

Shock

Shock is a common reaction to bad news, not an emotion in its own right. It's more useful to think of it as a state that the person experiences when one of several emotions is felt intensely and "supramaximally." Shock is a condition in which the person loses much of the normal decision-making ability and is basically unable to process the information he or she is being given (or much else). It is similar to the situation when the needle on a tape-recorder decibel meter shows that the sound coming in from the microphone is "peaking" or is being subjected to "overload." The recorder can't handle the input; there will be distortion (and perhaps even some form of longer-lasting damage).

The state of psychological shock is similar. It can happen to any of us; we can all become shocked by a sudden overload of fear, anxiety, anger, disappointment, or other emotions.

The important thing about shock in the clinical setting is that the patient often doesn't say, "I am shocked!" The patient may say, "Oh, my goodness," or, "Oh, dear," or just, "Oh." He or she may even say nothing at all but may simply stare back at you with a blank expression, a face that basically tells you, "I'm not handling this information."

When the patient is shocked, it is helpful for you to acknowledge that, even using simple phrases as in this example:

➤ *Situation:*
The patient has had three hours of retrosternal chest pain. The ECG shows a small inferior infarct. You tell the patient that.

> *The Patient Says:*
> "Oh, my god!"
> *You Can Choose From:*
> —*Direct or Factual Response*
>   "It's not that bad, really."
> —*Escalationary or Judgmental Response*
>   "Come on, relax a bit. Getting into a state will only make it
>   worse."
> —*Open Question*
>   "Tell me what's going through your mind."
> —*Empathic Response*
>   "This is obviously a big shock."

Fear

When the news is particularly bad, it is reasonable to expect fear as part of the patient's first reaction. In fact, if the news is unequivocally serious and the patient doesn't express any fear, your first thought should be, "Does this person understand what I'm saying?"

The important point is that when the patient expresses a fear, you should acknowledge it before going on—a few seconds later—to explore the particular objects of that fear and then to agree on a plan.

Here's a straightforward example of a patient expressing fear about a gastroscopy.

➤ *Situation:*

The patient has had intermittent epigastric pain over the last few months, with no weight loss, but with only slight improvement with the medication. You recommend a gastroscopy.

> *The Patient Says*
> "Oh, my gosh! I couldn't face something like that!"
> *You Can Choose From:*
> —*Direct or Factual Response*
> "It's only a little procedure. It takes a few minutes, that's all."
> —*Escalationary or Judgmental Response*
> "Come on, don't be a baby. It's nothing."
> —*Open Question*
> "What particularly makes you say that?"
> —*Empathic Response*
> "I realize this is scary for you. What's the biggest worry with a gastroscopy?"

Anger

Some people become angry over events that don't bother other people at all, so the rest of the world calls those people "angry people." It is not known exactly why and how individuals vary in their thresholds for anger, but it seems to be a fact of our species. We each have our own in-dividual threshold for anger, and not only does that threshold vary from person to person but also it varies with the circumstances. An event that may make us angry on a bleak dark Monday morning (e.g., traffic) may not trouble us at all on a sunny weekend. People who have a low thresh-old for expressions of anger most of the time are usually regarded as angry or grumpy individuals.

Looking after a habitually angry person who has a serious medical condition can be somewhat difficult. We cannot do much (if anything) about their *general* anger state, although we might be able to help them cope with particular impinging events. The secret is to try and identify the triggers or targets of the anger and to acknowledge the emotion and what they are experiencing—even if (as often happens) there is nothing fixable about it.

To start the process, here is a rough categorization of things that make people angry when they are ill.

Abstract Anger

Anger at the disease. Common targets include every type of physical symptom, including pain, loss of mobility, nausea, sleep disturbance, anorexia, fatigue, malaise, and so on, often amplified by loss of freedom and dependency on others.

Anger at loss of control and at powerlessness. Being dependant on others is extremely irritating and frustrating to many people, and being under the apparent control of the physicians and nurses is another facet of this.

Anger at loss of potential. Few of us have achieved all of the hopes and dreams that we once had! Loss of potential is a major source of irritation, and it usually increases as physical abilities wane.

Anger at randomness/laws of nature. The almost ubiquitous sense of unfairness is perhaps the major factor in "why me?"

Anger at Specific Entities

Anger at self. Many patients feel—often inappropriately—that they have caused their own condition. (For some reason, most patients with smoking-related cancers do not feel that or do not express it.) The emotion generated by this process is seen as guilt.

Anger at friends and family. Commonly, ancient family feuds and grudges are reignited during illness, and they are often made worse by the current good health of the family members (another example of the unfairness of the illness). These targets of anger may be more visible in cases including AIDS, sexually transmitted conditions, or conditions related to passive smoking, as well as in situations in which the patient feels abandoned.

Anger at members of the medical team. Anger directed at the doctors and nurses who are looking after the patient is common. It is partly due to the fact that we are there—and therefore act as lightning rods for the tension in the air. Other factors include loss of control, and resentment of the apparent health of the professionals and any gaps in communication (including not acknowledging emotions expressed by the patient).

Anger at outside agencies. Specific complaints are often precipitated by the employer, the insurance company, government agencies, reimbursements for medical expenses, and so on.

Anger at God. The depth and length of a person's previous religious faith may have nothing to do with their anger or resentment against apparent abandonment ("I've been forsaken") or against feared retribution in the afterlife (a reaction I have seen only once or twice, fueled by unhelpful doctrines and dogmas spread by small but forceful religious cults).

Dealing with Anger

The secret in dealing with anger is to acknowledge that it is an emotion and not to get drawn in—on one side or the other—of any "blame game."

The following example shows how you can address the emotion without a specific judgment when the target of the anger is the referring doctor.

➤ *Situation:*

The patient has had three months of cough, occasionally productive of colorless sputum. He recently had two episodes of hemoptysis, and bronchoscopy showed lung cancer.

The Patient Says:
"And my family doctor said it was just a bit of bronchitis! I'm going to sue him!"
You Can Choose From:
—*Direct or Factual Response*
  "Didn't he even do a chest x-ray?"
—*Escalationary or Judgmental Response*
  "Listen, if you're planning to sue him, you're not going to get any help from me."
—*Open Question*
  "Say more about those feelings."
—*Empathic Response*
  "You sound angry that this wasn't picked up earlier."

Disbelief

Disbelief is a common reaction to hearing bad news. As we've seen, the "badness" of bad news lies in the amount by which it lowers the person's expectations of the future. If that gap between expectations and reality is too large, it is difficult for the person to take in the information. This is why, in general, the patients who have the greatest difficulty are those who feel physically well at a time when the diagnosis is very serious (for ample, acute myeloid leukemia in a young, fit adult). By and large, when the person feels ill and has several symptoms, it is intellectually a little easier for them to take the information on board.

The important thing with disbelief is to acknowledge that the patient is experiencing it (with an empathic response) and not to direct your response simply to the facts of the matter.

➤ *Situation:*
The patient is a 65-year-old male whose prostate biopsies show a moderately differentiated cancer (Gleason score 3+4). You tell the patient that.

> *The Patient Says:*
> "Cancer? No, that's got to be a mistake."
> *You Can Choose From:*
> —*Direct or Factual Response*
>   "No, it isn't a mistake. It's definitely your biopsy."
> —*Escalationary or Judgmental Response*
>   "We don't make mistakes here."
> —*Open Question*
>   "What is it that makes you say that?"
> —*Empathic Response*
>   "I know this is difficult to believe."

Despair

When the other person is in despair, as health care professionals we usually have a strong urge to fix it, to dispel it, to cure and abolish it. However, that is not usually possible in one step. The secret with responding to an expression of despair is first to acknowledge its presence. No matter what your medical management plan is, it is crucial first to tell the patient that you can see that he or she is feeling that things are hopeless.

After acknowledging the patient's feelings at that moment, you can proceed to talk about the most significant factors precipitating the despair in the case, and subsequently you can agree on a plan of management. However, that will not work until after you have acknowledged the way the person is feeling at that moment.

Here's an example of how you might frame your first sentence or two.

➤ *Situation:*

The patient has non-small-cell lung cancer. It was partially responsive to chemotherapy and then biologics. It is now progressing and has not responded to the latest chemotherapy. You tell the patient that.

> *The Patient Says:*
> "Oh, that's terrible. Now I've got nothing to look forward to."
> *You Can Choose From:*
> —*Direct or Factual Response*
>   "Well, there's no further treatment for the cancer, but we can still look after any symptoms."
> —*Escalationary or Judgmental Response*
>   "Come on, you just have to look at the positive side—for example, not needing any more chemo."
> —*Open Question*
>   "What are you feeling right now?"
> —*Empathic Response*
>   "This is awful for you, isn't it? Tell me about the most worrying aspects."

Crying

Although many readers will know how to handle the situation when the other person begins to cry, a few guidelines are worth emphasizing.

1. *Offer a tissue.* When the other person is crying, there is no substitute for offering a tissue. If there isn't a box of tissues handy, then ask the patient if he or she has one handy. If not, it's worth leaving the

room to get one. For the patient, this gives him or her permission to cry and, of course, something to dab the tears with and something to partly hide behind. Further conversation is now possible and valuable; without a tissue, meaningful dialogue becomes awkward and almost impossible.

2. *Move closer, break eye contact, and (perhaps) touch the forearm.* Most people feel isolated when they cry. I have found it helpful to move closer to the person. At the same time, I break eye contact (so it doesn't seem as if I'm staring) and usually position myself ninety degrees to them and gently and briefly touch the back of the person's forearm. Some people—including some doctors—don't like physical contact, so if you are not comfortable doing it, don't. Similarly, if the patient draws away from you, don't make physical contact again.

3. *Keep silent for a moment.* When the other person cries, there is no need to say anything for a few seconds. That silence in itself shows that you do not disapprove of his or her crying, and you are therefore giving a nonjudgmental response.

4. *Ask an open question about the immediate cause of the crying.* Ideally, your first response when the other person cries should be to ask the person to try to say what particularly precipitated the tears. In other words, the ideal response to crying is to explore the immediate cause of it.

➤ *Situation:*
The patient has had difficulty walking for a few weeks. An MRI shows multiple demyelinating plaques. The diagnosis of multiple sclerosis is explained to the patient.

> *The Patient Says:*
> (The patient looks shocked for a second, then begins to cry.)
> *You Can Choose From:*
> —*Direct or Factual Response*
>   "Here's what we're going to do . . ."
> —*Escalationary or Judgmental Response*
>   "Come on, don't cry. You've got to face this positively."
> —*Open Question*
>   "What's the most painful part of that right now?"

—*Empathic Response*
   (Offering a tissue) "This is painful and shocking, isn't it?"

"Why Me?"

"Why me?" is not really a question; it is a statement of an emotion that includes despair, which may have several sources. The important thing is to find out what triggered the "Why me?" at this particular moment—and that means you should ask.

➤ *Situation:*
   The patient presented with an atypical mycobacterium infection and has just been diagnosed as having AIDS.

   The Patient Says:
   "AIDS! Oh, my god! Why me?"
   You Can Choose From:
   —*Direct or Factual Response*
      "You knew the risks you were taking."
   —*Escalationary or Judgmental Response*
      "Well, that's what you get from taking those kinds of risks."
   —*Open Question*
      "What's going through your mind at the moment?"
   —*Empathic Response*
      "It's really tough, isn't it?"
      NB: The empathic response here sidesteps the apparent question form of the phrase "Why me?" and treats it solely as a cry of suffering.

Depression

Depression is a constant feeling of low spirits and lack of any feelings of happiness—plus a few other features—lasting outside the "normal" range for that person, and being present for most of the time for at least two weeks.

In table 2.5, I've slightly paraphrased the DSM-IV criteria to make it easier for you to use as a guideline.

TABLE 2.5   *A Practical Guide to the Diagnosis of Depression*

A person is clinically depressed if five of the following features have been present, and outside the person's usual range of feelings, for most of the time over a period of two weeks with no other apparent cause. One of the symptoms must be 1 or 2.

1. Feeling low in spirits, feeling depressed
2. Nothing makes the person feel happy or joyful (anhedonia) or interested
3. Disordered appetite (loss of appetite or overeating) with weight gain or loss when there is no other cause
4. Disordered sleep patterns (inability to get to sleep or early wakening and inability to get to sleep again)
5. Disordered bodily activity, feeling sluggish and unable to do normal activities or overactive and unable to keep still
6. Exhaustion, fatigue, feeling tired all the time
7. Feelings of worthlessness, low self-esteem, self-loathing
8. Being unable to concentrate, unable to focus or hold focus
9. Thoughts about death or dying, thoughts of suicide

➤ *Situation:*

A 52-year-old man has diabetes, which is well controlled. He recently lost his job.

> *The Patient Says:*
> "I just feel so miserable all the time."
> *You Can Choose From:*
> —*Direct or Factual Response*
>   "That's something we can fix with the right medication."
> —*Escalationary or Judgmental Response*
>   "You've got to buck up a bit, you know."
> —*Open Question*
>   "How bad are those feelings?"
> —*Empathic Response*
>   "You sound really low in your spirits."

Displacement and "The Quest"

Many people respond to bad news by immediately deciding on an activity or task to which they commit themselves. There are probably many reasons for doing this. First, it may be something that is valuable to the community (large or small) and therefore makes the person feel valuable and—if the task can be completed—valued. In other words, it may genuinely be a worthwhile project. In addition, it has value to the person because it gives her or him an additional focus of activity and thought and thus may distract the person from dwelling on the feelings associated with the medical condition.

The project may also be a form of bargaining. If there is, let us say, only a small chance of the person surviving longer than two years and the person plans a project to be carried out over five years, it becomes a disguised bargaining process between the person and destiny. ("I'll do this worthwhile thing if you'll allow me to live for five years.")

For all these reasons, then, what is termed *displacement behavior* may form a functioning part of the patient's coping strategy. Because such activity might be useful—even if only as a temporary measure—it is important to acknowledge that and to try hard not to be judgmental. Even if you think that the goals are simply not feasible, you can still reinforce the value of the effort from the patient's viewpoint.

➤ *Situation:*

The patient has an incurable neurological condition similar to Lou Gehrig's disease. He decides to raise funds and start a regular international conference of researchers to try and find the cure.

The Patient Says:
"I'm going to do this! And we're going to find the cure."
You Can Choose From:
—*Direct or Factual Response*
"I don't think that's possible. Research has been going on for thirty years with nothing major yet."
—*Escalationary or Judgmental Response*
"Oh, right: the world is just waiting for you to solve the puzzle."
—*Open Question*
"What are you hoping for?"
—*Empathic Response*
"You are clearly full of energy and commitment, which is good for you and may also be good for other people with this condition. The process sounds helpful."

After acknowledging the patient's commitment and energy, you can go on to discuss the points mentioned above—that the quest will give a new focus to the person and is far better than simply allowing the anxieties to affect mood and energy. Even if you are thinking to yourself, "This scheme has no chance of achieving its objectives," you can replace that in your own mind with something like, "This scheme—even if it doesn't achieve its goals—might turn out to be a beneficial part of this person's coping strategies."

As has often been said, a belief doesn't have to be true to make the believer feel better.

Humor

Humor is a coping strategy that many—but not all—people use to reduce the magnitude of a threat. When it is used—and understood—as a mechanism for coping with the bad news, it can be valuable and can be a major part of the patient's repertoire of adaptive responses.

Hence, if your patient does make a light-hearted comment about a grim subject, provided that the person clearly has understood the gravity of the news, you can—and should—respond to the tone and reinforce it so that the person feels rewarded for having made that type of an effort.

It is important to realize that responding to a patient's humor is not the same as initiating it yourself. Although there has been a lot of discussion prompted by books[3] and movies[4] about humor as having an effect on the disease, there are (so far) no data to support that hypothesis. At the moment, then, humor is an important part of the way many humans communicate with each other, but it doesn't seem to have any direct effect on disease processes.

Therefore, I strongly recommend *not* "inflicting humor" on the patient, although you can (and perhaps should) acknowledge and respond to it (as in the example below). Humor seems to be a valuable lubricant of human communication and can be used *after* a serious discussion about the serious issues—but *never instead of* it.

➤ *Situation:*
You have just explained that the patient's condition is serious and the chance of it responding to treatment is only about 30 percent.

The Patient Says:
"Oh, well. It's lucky I've got a good insurance plan for my widow."
You Can Choose From:
—*Direct or Factual Response*
   "Yes, that's good. Let's hope it won't be used."
—*Escalationary or Judgmental Response*
   "This is no time to make light of a serious matter."
—*Open Question*
   "What particularly were you thinking of when you said that?"
—*Empathic Response*
   "That's a philosophical way of looking at it. It's a tough way to get money out of insurance companies, though."

Families and Their Reactions

The important thing to remember about dealing with a family—or a circle of family members or friends—is that you probably have no real idea of the relationships between the members. Fortunately, that ignorance won't stop you from doing a reasonable job in communicating with that patients' circle.

You don't have to be some kind of superpsychiatrist or be able to analyze and understand all of the wrinkles and nuances in your patient's relationships with the rest of the group to be able to help and reinforce the support system.

Dissonance

In families it is common to find people who have very different views and opinions from those of the patient. For example, the patient may have decided that since third-line chemotherapy had no effect on the cancer, he is not willing to try fourth-line. By contrast, the patient's wife may strongly want him to try it. ("You can't give up now, George. You've got to try it.")

You don't have to be the referee choosing one side to the exclusion of the other. Rather, you can give support to both parties.

Supporting the Family Member and the Patient

Fortunately for us, as health care professionals, the ethical guidelines governing our practice are relatively unequivocal: a mentally competent patient has the right to decide on his or her own treatment. If there is any type of dispute about treatment, the patient's own wishes (if mental competency is not in question) have primacy.

Now, that is, as it were, the "bottom line." It tells you whose rights have priority if push comes to shove. But far more important is the task of trying to prevent pushing and shoving.

The secret here is to realize that most families (as well as the patients they gather around) are scared. You will often see anger or frenetic overactivity, interference, bossiness, emotional roller coasters, tears, bargaining, and pleading, even complaints and legal action. At the root of most of this is almost always fear, combined with a desire to "make it all right" for the patient.

Once you realize that this fear is usually the emotional state underlying most of the actions, you can acknowledge it, which usually will reduce the aggression and opposition considerably.

➤ *Situation:*
The patient is in his late 60s and has non-small-cell lung cancer, progressing after the first chemotherapy regimen. He is asymptomatic, and second-line chemotherapy would extend his survival by a short time only, if at all.

The Relative Says:
"My brother's simply *got* to have the next type of chemotherapy."
You Can Choose From:
—*Direct or Factual Response*
   "No, he hasn't got to have it. The decision is his and his alone."
—*Escalationary or Judgmental Response*
   "I can't give it to him simply on your say-so—but I could give it to *you* instead!"
—*Open Question*
   "What is going through your mind right now?"
—*Empathic Response*
   "I know you want the best for your brother. And in our own way, we all do. But even though you clearly want the best for him, this is a time when *his* own wishes count."

"My Mother's Not to Be Told"

Perhaps one of the most common conflicts within families when it comes to breaking bad news is the instruction—sometimes made forcibly—that "my mother is not to be told how serious her situation is." The difficulty of the "my mother's not to be told" situation is that the rights of the patient are clear, but the needs and concerns of the relative are also important and need at least to be acknowledged.

The rights of the patient—in terms of legal, moral, and ethical issues—are now well established. In almost all countries, organizations, and situations, the mentally competent patient has the paramount right to receive any medical information about his or her condition. Equally, the patient has the right *not* to hear that information if that is what she or he desires. In other words, the patient may abrogate her or his right to that information.

The dilemma is that the relative is *telling* you on behalf of his or her mother that this is what she wants, and almost invariably the relative is a significant part of the patient's support circle and is important to the patient. Hence it would be good to avoid an all-out confrontation with the relative.

It might help if you look at scenario 6 on the accompanying DVD, in which you will see how you can handle this situation. In this scenario, the son of a woman who is a new patient with a breast lump, comes into the consultation room before the patient has been seen and insists that, if the lump is a cancer, his mother is not to be told.

Clearly, the patient has the ethical and legal right to hear the information if she wants to know it, but—equally clearly—the relative wants to protect his mother from the shock of what appears to be harmful information. Furthermore, it is likely that the son plays a part in the patient's support system. In the particular situation in scenario 6, the son is the translator because his mother speaks only Gujarati. In any event, even if the relative were not the most available translator, it would be ill advised to simply overrule him and thus try to cut him out of the circle of support.

The key of the strategic approach in this situation is to acknowledge clearly the son's laudable and appropriate motive in wanting to protect his mother. At the same time, however, it is important to stay firm on the principle that his mother has the right to that information if she wants it.

I have found that it works well if you arrange with the son to have an interview with the mother *with the son present* so that you can ask her a question to the effect "If your test results turn out to be something serious, would you like to know what's going on in detail?" If you are using the son as the translator, it helps to ask him to translate her reply honestly and faithfully.

(On the matter of medicolegal procedures, it is important to record the result of that conversation in the chart, even if it is only one sentence: "The patient has indicated through her son as translator that she does not want to know the diagnosis but would like all information to be given to him.")

You can see how this strategy can be made to work as illustrated in scenario 6, but here are the various options that could be followed, set out in the "crossroads" format.

➤ *Situation:*
The patient is a 70-year-old Gujarati-speaking woman whom you have not yet met. Before you see her, her son bursts into the consultation room.

> *The Son Says:*
> "If it's cancer, you are not to tell my mother."
> *You Can Choose From:*
> —*Direct or Factual Response*
>   "I have to tell her. It's her right."
> —*Escalationary or Judgmental Response*
>   "Nobody tells me what goes into—or doesn't go into—a conversation between doctor and patient."
> —*Open Question*
>   "What do you mean when you say that?"
> —*Empathic Response*
>   "You are obviously worried about your mother. What's the most worrying thing about this?"

In this discussion it is important to affirm the son's importance as part of his mother's support but to establish clearly that his mother's rights to information have precedence over the son's wishes. In other words, even if the son does not wish his mother to have that information, the mother is the patient and she has the right to be told that information *if* she wants it, and also has the right not to be told, if that is what she wants.

Talking with Children

Talking with children can be tricky, whether they are the children of your patient or are the patients themselves. From my limited experience in pediatric oncology and my more extensive practice dealing with the children of adult oncology patients, I have come to discern four constant principles in talking with children (meaning teenagers or younger).

Whenever possible, have the parent or caregiver present. I think it advisable to have the parent or caregiver present when you are talking with the child, unless that is impossible. If for some reason it is not possible, then at least try to get a message through to the parent and say that you will talk with him or her about the interview at a later date.

Communicate at the level of the child's understanding (not chronological age). For those of us who are not pediatricians, we might harbor the belief that we should talk to the child at a level appropriate to their chronological age. But chronological age is an unreliable guiding principle. You may find yourself talking to a canny and wise 11 year old who is able to see the whole situation or to a 14 year old who does not see the bigger picture. The important thing is to try to match the level of your vocabulary to the level of the other person's understanding. Generally, it is probably better to start with words with ordinary meaning such as "serious" or phrases such as "will take a few weeks to get better," and so on. It is always easier to raise the level of your vocabulary during the conversation than to lower it (which usually seems patronizing).

Be prepared to repeat what you say. Depending on their level of understanding, younger children may ask you to repeat the message several times. It may seem at first as if the other person is deliberately needling you, but that isn't the reason. Children often want to hear you say the same thing two or three times simply to be sure that you mean it. Children often do that with parents and adults at home: "Do you *really* mean you want me to go to bed before eleven?"

If you are not used to talking with children, do be aware of this need for repetition, and try to be more patient than you would be with an adult doing the same thing. Time spent in reinforcing the message and in making empathic responses to what the child is experiencing is a good investment.

Remember magical thinking. Magical thinking is what happens when a child (or anyone!) believes that something he or she has done or failed to do—or even thought about—has caused an event. ("Mom told me to tidy my room and I didn't, so now she's ill and needs an operation.") It may seem obvious to us that the child's not doing a household chore has nothing to do with the parent's medical condition, but sometimes making a connection between those two events is how children think. Hence, it is worthwhile stating clearly when talking to children that the condition is not their fault.

Of course, there is much more to communicating with children than these four simple guidelines, but if you do not customarily talk with children, you may find it helpful to keep these simple principles in mind.

2.5. Some Useful Strategies in Discussing the Prognosis in Terminal Illness

Almost everybody—doctors and patients alike—finds it difficult to talk about dying and imminent death. There are many reasons for this (which I have discussed at length elsewhere).[5]

"How Long Do I Have?"

Many times in your career, a patient will ask you how long he or she has.

There are four useful guidelines in handling this difficult question:

1. CLARIFY AND ACKNOWLEDGE

It's often worth restating the question "Would you like me to try to estimate how long you have to live?" Sometimes that won't be needed; you do not need to clarify if the patient clearly asks, "How long have I got to live?" But occasionally when the patient says something like, "How long?" he or she actually means something quite different, such as "How long will it be before I can return to work?" In all situations, it is always worth acknowledging that this is a difficult and important question (i.e., make an empathic response).

2. DON'T GIVE AN EXACT FIGURE

Because you will be wrong! Physicians have been shown to be consistently overoptimistic when they estimate the prognosis (compared to both nurses and relatives).[6] Even so, you do have an ethical obligation to try to answer the question, so perhaps giving a general estimate is what you should do.

3. DO GIVE A REASONABLE BALLPARK ESTIMATE OF HOW MUCH TIME THE PATIENT HAS

Patients have a right to know how long they will survive in general terms, and they may have no idea of the situation. Patients who have a low-grade lymphoma may think they'll be dead before next Christmas (whereas the median survival in many series is longer than seven years). On the other hand, a young mother of two who has advanced small-cell lung cancer might think that she has at least five years ahead of her (whereas the chance of that happening is less than 5 percent).

Here are some phrases that I often use which may be helpful:

- "It'll probably be several years. Not decades, but several years."
- "It's likely to be a small number of years or a large number of months."
- "It's most likely that we're taking about several months: probably many, but it could be a small number."
- "We're probably looking at several weeks or a small number of months."
- "Unfortunately, we're probably looking at a few weeks only."
- "We're probably looking at less than a week."

4. ACKNOWLEDGE THE UNCERTAINTY

Most people find the state of uncertainty—of "not knowing what the answer is"—highly unpleasant.

Nowadays most of us are accustomed to having a high degree of control over most aspects of our life (what to wear and eat, where to go for relaxation, what to watch or listen to, and so on). Against that background, the uncertainty of a serious medical condition is jarring and deeply disturbing. Often in clinical practice you simply will be unable to tell the person how the condition is going to respond or progress in the immediate future. That uncertainty is extremely unpleasant, and it may even erode the patient's trust in your clinical abilities. You can support the patient and to some extent reverse that distrust by clearly acknowledging the unpleasantness of uncertainty. It is a valuable empathic response that you will find you use often.

➤ *Situation:*

The patient has pancreatic cancer, which has recurred and is progressing after a response to gemcitabine.

> *The Patient Says:*
> "How long am I going to live?"
> *You Can Choose From:*
> —*Direct or Factual Response*
>   "Two months. Three at best."
> —*Escalationary or Judgmental Response*
>   "I don't have a crystal ball. Nobody knows how long you have."
> —*Open Question*
>   "Tell me what you've been thinking."
> —*Empathic Response*
>   "That's obviously an important question for you."

In my own practice, I commonly combine an empathic response with an open question. So if I don't know the patient—or the recent events—very well, I might say, "That's a major issue for you, of course. Why don't you tell me what you think?"

It's worth your looking at scenario 4 on the DVD to see how it is possible to elicit the patient's perception of the situation and then to show him that his own attitude to risk management must be the main deciding factor in the treatment plan.

Hope: The Positive and the Negative

In some respects, we are always treading a fine line between telling the truth, which may be cold and hard, and painting an overoptimistic picture of the future, which will be easier on both parties for a short time but will not allow the patient to make appropriate plans.

There are two central issues here: (1) hope, if is based on an unrealistic basis, can be an "enemy" rather than a friend, and (2) hope is not one single monolithic entity but has many components, many of which might be realizable while some are not.

Unrealistic Hope: A Potential Enemy

The Cornell physician and author Eric Cassell expressed the potentially damaging effects of unrealistic hope in the following analogy (which I have paraphrased slightly):

> Imagine that I am trying to catch the 8 A.M. flight to Toronto. I'm running late, and at 8 A.M. instead of sitting on board the plane, I am running down the concourse toward the gate. Am I crazy to be running? Perhaps not, because sometimes flights are delayed for ten minutes and people can still get on board a couple of minutes after the scheduled departure time (as actually happened this morning). Also in my pocket I have the kind of ticket that can be changed to another flight and I have access to the timetable of flights on the Internet with my BlackBerry. So I wouldn't be thought of as crazy to be running.
>
> But what if I was due to catch the 8 A.M. flight and I am running down the concourse for the 8 A.M. flight at 11 A.M.? Or 2 P.M.? Or the following day? And what if my ticket is nonrefundable, so I can't change it if I miss the flight? And what if I have no way of finding out about other flights? Would I be thought of as crazy then? Probably.[7]

The point here is important: *What* you do is less important than *how* you have planned the alternatives. This is why the tactic of "plan for the worst and hope for the best" (see below) is so valuable (though many people like to reverse the order of those phrases).

Another analogy that I have heard (and sometimes use) compares hope and planning with getting ready to pay income tax. If a person makes regular installment payments toward the estimated income tax bill and knows that there is enough money in the current account to meet any shortfall, then that person has made a realistic plan. By contrast, another person, when asked what plans he or she has made for paying the taxes, might reply: "Oh, I've bought a lottery ticket. I have a feeling that I'm going to win." We could say that, in the latter case, hope is getting in the way of organizing proper plans. As Cassell might say, hope is acting, in some senses, as an enemy.

Our job is made easier when we explore the plan-and-still-hope strategy. Furthermore, it is easier to discuss plans for deterioration and even death when those discussions are held early, before they are required.

"Can You Cure Me?"

Often (particularly in oncology), the patient's greatest wish—complete permanent resolution (i.e., cure) of the condition—may simply not be achievable. In all areas of medicine it often happens that the patient most of all wants a cure for a condition that is incurable. If such a cure is not one of the options, then you can still explain the plan in terms of dealing with *some* of the patient's wishes.

The following situation is an example, and I deal with additional responses in the section on Wish Statements below.

➤ *Situation:*
  The patient has breast cancer, which has now spread.

  The Patient Says:
  "You can still cure me, can't you?"
  You Can Choose From:
  —*Direct or Factual Response*
    "Sadly, that's not possible."
  —*Escalationary or Judgmental Response*
    "I'm not Superman, you know."
  —*Open Question*
    "Tell me what you mean when you say *cure*."
  —*Empathic Response*
    "I know that's what you want, but unfortunately it's simply not possible in this situation."

The Use of "Wish Statements"

There is nothing wrong with making "wish statements"—saying straightforwardly and directly what you would like to see happen. Doing so achieves many things. It shows the patient that you—as a person—would want certain things (usually the same things as the patient wants!) and that even you, as a professional, cannot produce these things, although you wish it were possible.

Furthermore, once you have used a wish statement, you can then go on to describe those things that you *can* do. Hence, you have acknowledged what is *not* possible, as a preface to reinforcing the things that *are* possible.

➤ *Situation:*
The patient is about to have pelvic surgery for stage III ovarian carcinoma.

> *The Patient Says:*
> "Give me your guarantee that the operation will fix the problem. Please."
> *You Can Choose From:*
> —*Direct or Factual Response*
>   "That's not possible."
> —*Escalationary or Judgmental Response*
>   "Come on, be realistic."
> —*Open Question*
>   "Tell me what's going through your mind."
> —*Empathic Response*
>   "I realize this is a big worry for you."
> —*Wish Statement*
>   "I wish I could guarantee that. I *can* guarantee that I will do my best, and if all of it can be removed, I'll do it."

In my own practice, I am likely to make an empathic response first, immediately followed by a wish statement. ("I know that's what you want, and it's what I want, too, but I can't guarantee that result right now. All I *can* guarantee is that . . .")

Plan for the Worst / Hope for the Best

In this section, I talk about progressive disease, when the prognosis is limited—in other words, situations in which the patient is expected to die in the foreseeable future.

Obviously, these are extremely difficult conversations to hold, and entire books have been written about just such situations. Hence, what I am about to outline is the briefest of summaries. If palliative and end-of-life care is a major feature of your own practice, I suggest that it's worth reading one of the textbooks on the subject (especially if I am the author on the chapter about communication!).[8]

The point that needs emphasis is this: the human mind is capable of planning for the worst while still hoping for the best.

Furthermore, as mentioned above, it is easier to make plans for the end of life before they are needed. It is much more difficult to make those plans and arrangements when events are happening fast and there is a sense of urgency.

For those reasons, I strongly recommend that if you have a patient who is not doing well, you broach the subject of dying and discuss the arrangements that the patient would like *before* those things are needed. Furthermore, the atmosphere is a little easier if the arrangements that you discuss are—to a certain extent—hypothetical and are not a set of decisions that need to be made this minute.

There is another big advantage of making plans for the worst eventuality. Making those plans gives the patient at least some feeling of control over events or at least over his or her responses to those events.

This idea was perhaps best phrased by the Viennese psychiatrist Viktor Frankl in his 1948 book, *Man's Search for Meaning*. Having survived the Nazi concentration camps, Frankl had come to the conclusion that everything can be taken away from you except your choice of how you react to the events. This is a brilliant and perceptive thought, and I often refer to Frankl (at the right moment and in the right atmosphere) when talking about these things with my patients.

For all those reasons, then, although the issues are intrinsically difficult, the discussions can be made a little easier when you use this plan-and-still-hope strategy. Here's an example of how it can be used in conjunction with an empathic response.

➤ *Situation:*
The patient has non-small-cell lung cancer, which has now progressed on third-line chemotherapy. There are no further therapy options for treating the cancer.

The Patient Says:

"I'm not going to die of this, am I?"

You Can Choose From:

—*Direct or Factual Response*

"Well, you're not dying now."

—*Escalationary or Judgmental Response*

"Don't talk like that."

—*Open Question*

"What's going through your mind at the moment?"

—*Empathic Response*

"I know this is difficult. But perhaps it will help if we talk about planning for the worst, which won't stop any of us from hoping for the best. Tell me what the big issues are."

2.6. Summary: Asking before Telling Helps the Interview Start Well

Sharing bad news is never easy. It may be devastating for the patient, and it challenges any ideas that we may have about being able to "fix it" every time. The importance of the SPIKES protocol is that you obtain the patient's perceptions before you give the information. Before you tell, ask. Then respond to the patient's emotions as they arise.

The CONES Protocol for Disclosing Error

		Topics covered in this chapter
C	**C**ontext	Setting. Greeting.
O	**O**pening remark	Set the agenda immediately and briefly. Don't be afraid of saying *sorry*.
N	**N**arrative	Explain major events in chronological (narrative) order, responding to emotions and questions.
E	**E**motions	Acknowledge the emotions expressed.
S	**S**trategy and **S**ummary	Strategy must include quick follow-up (hours?). Summary must include contact and other personnel.

CHAPTER THREE

Disclosing Error

The CONES Protocol

....

An example of "when you have to tell"

As we have just seen, in the sharing of bad news, it is helpful to find out what the patient already knows before asking whether he or she would like you to discuss the news. By contrast, when there has been a medical error, in most situations you will be obliged to tell the patient about it, whether he or she overtly wants to hear it or not.

In those circumstances—as well as in other situations in which you have to tell, such as informing a relative of the death or of a sudden deterioration in the patient's medical state—you will find that the CONES strategy is well suited. (You can see an example of how this approach works in clinical practice in scenario 7 on the accompanying DVD.)

As a preface to that protocol, let us begin with a brief general overview of the error disclosure.

3.1. Errors Happen! The "Blame Culture" versus "System Failure" Analysis

....

There is no human system in which errors do not occur.

Fifty years ago, disclosing an error was frowned on and almost forbidden. Of course, both doctors and patients accepted that errors occurred, but the medicolegal environment originating in the United States created an atmosphere in which physicians strenuously avoided open discussion of error, fearing that it would lead to punitive damages (which it often did) as well as to deleterious effects on career and reputation.

Today's atmosphere is different. Perhaps one of the most important signs of that is a paper by the Veterans Administration published a few years ago in which error disclosure was initially carried out by a member of the administrative staff and resulted in the hospital paying out a lower dollar amount of compensation (although the number of cases resulting in a legal suit rose slightly). This result was widely regarded as showing that honesty and error disclosure were good things for the hospital to embrace. The lower dollar amount paid out in settlement was regarded as indicating a greater degree of satisfaction.[1] Further studies supporting the same general conclusion and its neutral or even beneficial effect on litigation and costs have been published more recently.[2]

Even so, as several authors have pointed out,[3] the medical profession has developed relatively few mechanisms for preventing and disclosing error, when compared to other high-profile industries, such as the airline industry, for example.

The medicolegal principle ruling medical error in the past was straightforward, but its limitations had unhelpful results. If an error occurred, even if the patient sustained no harm as a result, the physician and/or the hospital or institution would be held responsible and were liable for financial and other damages. This "culture of blame and shame" created an atmosphere in which little attention was given to learning from errors and subsequently modifying existing systems and/or creating new ones to prevent future repetitions of the same error.

Things have changed considerably over the last decade or so, and there is currently a much greater tendency to make a genuine effort at system analysis, to find out what part of the system allowed the error to occur, and to prevent it in the future.

The important thing about the process of failure analysis is that you have to acknowledge the person's condition and feelings as well as reveal the error. In other words, in discussing error you have to aim for two objectives in the same interview: (1) acknowledging the person's situation and feelings and (2) identifying (as far as is possible) how the error occurred and also how the system can be modified to prevent a future reoccurrence of the error.

As you will see, the CONES approach does facilitate both of those aims, which are incorporated in the E for Emotion step and the S for Strategy step.

The Advantages of Disclosure

Perhaps the most significant feature of disclosing error is that nowadays, in many institutions, it is the law to do so. Most of us are obliged legally to disclose significant errors whether we want to or not, regardless of any controversy about the morals or the ethics in the situation, and, in places where it isn't the law, it is usually mandated in the institution's regulations.

As mentioned above in the landmark paper on behalf of the Veterans Administration, it was clearly shown that when disclosure of error was given—in this study, an administrator rather than the physician gave it—the cost in dollars was considerably decreased. But perhaps the major advantage of honest and sensitive disclosure is in the way the doctor-patient relationship survives and may strengthen. I don't want to make too much of this, but the alternative—of concealing a significant error and hoping that it is not discovered—is a problem.

3.2. The Biggest Obstacle to Disclosing an Error Often Is Not Knowing How

Currently, there is an atmosphere in which full disclosure of significant error is encouraged and, in many places, mandatory.

The principle is becoming universal, but unfortunately the methodology is way behind. We have not yet developed any standardized methods of error disclosure. We know that we want to do it, but we aren't yet agreed on how.

In this setting, the CONES protocol may be useful because at least it offers a systematic approach to this awkward situation and furthermore offers some suggestions for dealing with the patients' and relatives' responses to distressing events.

3.3. Who Should Disclose the Error?

Like it or not, the disclosure of a medical error is almost always a high-profile event. Even if it does not start off like that, it has the potential for quickly becoming a significant event.

For that reason, I suggest that disclosure of error should be made at a *high level* within the team hierarchy of that *patient's care*. Preferably, it should be done by someone who has continuing responsibility for the patient and ongoing involvement in his or her care—someone whom the patient would consider to be "my doctor."

If at all possible, then, the disclosure in a hospital or institution setting should be made by a staff physician, someone who clearly has some share in the responsibility for the care of that patient. In some hospitals, it is specified that for serious incidents, the head of the hospital (usually an administrator but often a person who has an M.D. as well) should make the disclosure. This approach can work well in many circumstances, provided that it doesn't entail much delay. If that system is set up and is operational, it also has certain other advantages; the head of the hospital may well be experienced in these matters. Furthermore, it demonstrates to the patient or relative (and to any legal representatives, if it comes to that) that the hospital is taking the matter seriously.

However, there are also clear advantages to the disclosure being made by an identifiable person ("my doctor") in terms of the continuing relationship between the family and the medical team.

Overall, there probably isn't one single answer that addresses every possible situation, but thinking about this issue is worth the investment of time and effort.

3.4. The CONES Protocol

What makes the disclosure of error different from most other forms of bad news, then, is that it is inappropriate to offer the patient the option of having you disclose the information, as in the SPIKES protocol. (It would be equally inappropriate to obtain their perception of the situation. Clearly, it would be absurd to say something like, "When you came here to this hospital, did you think that we would give you the correct dose of medication or not?")

With error disclosure, the onus is on you to tell the patient (or family members)—whether or not there has been any harm caused. Hence, unlike the SPIKES protocol, the CONES protocol does not hinge on the "before you tell, ask" principle but offers a relatively steady way of proceeding to impart difficult information.

C: Context

In the difficult situation of disclosing error, the physical context of the interview is extremely important. More than ever, this is the situation in which it helps to get the physical factors as conducive as possible to good communication. So shake hands at the outset, introduce yourself, and sit down so that your eyes are on the same level as the other person's. Even though you are almost certainly not *feeling* relaxed, do try to *appear* relatively calm. If you are unsure of what to do, put your feet flat on the ground with your knees together and your hands palm downward on your lap, which at least looks relatively tranquil. (See table 3.1.)

O: Opening Remark

The opening remark is crucial.

All you need to do is to set the scene, to establish the agenda. In these trying circumstances, I must admit that I often use phrases that make me feel comfortable, so something like, "I'd like to talk to you about what's been going on in the last few hours," or "I'd like to discuss your mother's current condition and what has been going on," or words that produce the same effect.

The important thing about the opening remark is that at the start of the discussion you are demonstrating that you are ready to focus on recent serious events.

Should You Say "Sorry" First?

If the patient (or relative) has already been informed of the situation (for example, if they are relatives or parents of the patient to whom something serious has happened), it is helpful to use *sorry* as your opening word. In many recent cases, relatives have said overtly that the word *sorry* was what they most wanted to hear, and in some cases they pursued the case legally until they received an apology.

Many heads of departments or hospitals where high-profile cases of error have occurred say that they would encourage anyone in this situation to use the word *sorry* at the start of the interview. So there is nothing wrong with using it. As I explained when talking about the difficulties in

TABLE 3.1   *A Few Basic Tips*

Technique	Central Feature	Notes
Greeting	Use the person's name.	A simple way of establishing the "person" as well as the "problem"
Introduce yourself	Briefly say who you are and what you do.	Merely courteous
Shake hands	Make actual contact.	Don't do that if you have a cold.
Sit down!	Bring your eyes to the same level as the other person's.	Essential
Don't be too far away	Have less than four feet of space between you.	The optimal distance varies with gender and culture, but three feet is rarely wrong.
Adopt a neutral body posture	Look relaxed, or at least not too anxious or irritated.	Even if you don't feel relaxed (and most of us don't at these times), try to adopt the neutral body posture and look relaxed.
Lean forward	Don't sit back all the way against the chair.	Studies show that patients recognize this as a sign of being interested in them.
Be ready to smile	Smiling may not be your usual "thing," but it helps if you can manage it.	If you do smile, try to "smile with your whole face."
Switch on your listening skills	Silence and repetition	Consciously maintain silence as the patient starts talking. Then in your first sentence of response use a word or phrase from the patient's last sentence.

breaking bad news, the word *sorry* has two distinct meanings. It can be an expression of sympathy ("I am sorry for you") or a statement of regret with an implication of responsibility, as when we ordinarily say, "Oops, sorry." Because of this ambiguity, I tend to be a bit more careful than usual about the words that I use. Often, I will start the interview (as I am shaking hands) with "I'm sorry about this." This phrase, in itself, conveys some sympathy and is ambiguous enough to allow the conversation that follows to range over the events without ruling out (or including) personal responsibility immediately.

What matters is what follows that opening: explaining the sequence of events, while answering questions and identifying and acknowledging the person's feelings during the conversation.

N: Narrative

Having established the reason for and the content of this conversation, then you can proceed with explaining the events.

In doing this, you should try to achieve two objectives concurrently: (1) giving a logical chronological account of the events (the *narrative*), and (2) stopping and responding to any emotions or any questions that the other person produces as you explain the events (*questions and reactions*).

So, start at the beginning of the condition that has led to the current situation, and check as you go along that this accords with the patient's/relative's perception. ("Your mother has breast cancer that is quite aggressive, and that's why we decided on the stronger chemotherapy.")

1. ANSWER QUESTIONS AS TRUTHFULLY AS POSSIBLE

In this situation, it is important to be as truthful as possible. It is helpful to you to provide a narrative, including the way the situation looked *at the time*. For example, you might say, "When you came into the ER, we thought that the chest pain was coming from your heart. In other words, we thought that you'd had a small heart attack. That's why we did the ECG. Now, the ECG was normal—no heart attack—but we wanted those blood tests to see if there had been some damage to the heart but it was too small to show up on the ECG. Is this making sense so far?"

2. ADMIT WHEN YOU DON'T KNOW—AND OUTLINE YOUR PLAN FOR PROBLEM SOLVING

When you don't know, you are allowed to say, "I don't know"—but always go on to say how you are going to tackle the problem of finding out: "We don't know yet whether this particular bug will respond to these particular antibiotics, but we may have the answer by this evening or perhaps tomorrow morning. I'll ask the microbiology department what we know about the bug by the end of today, and I'll call you with what they say."

This sort of communication is often called advocacy, and it makes a big difference. In essence, it is the significant difference between simply saying, "I don't know," and saying, "I don't now but I'm going to do X in time frame Y to try to find out."

This type of advocacy—particularly in the context of error disclosure —is courteous and kind and tells the patient or relative of your commitment to sorting out the situation. It makes the patient or relative feel that you and he or she are on the same page.

3. ALWAYS ACCEPT THAT THE PROGNOSIS MAY BE GRAVE

If death is even remotely possible, then it is a good idea to say that. As regards the outcome, it is usually better to have discussions about the worst-case scenario—and it is easier to hold those conversations earlier rather than later so that what you are discussing is the possibility of the worst-case scenario.

Most of us find it somewhat difficult to talk about a patient deteriorating and dying following an error. However, there are two things to remember in this situation:

1. It's usually better to talk about the worst possibilities early. (This has the added advantage that if things stabilize or improve, your clinical skills will be credited for the upturn.)
2. You can always frame an empathic response to your own discomfort; for example, "It's difficult talking about deteriorating or dying— it's difficult for me as well—but it may be better to talk about these things anyway."

You'll see how that possibility is handled in scenario 7 on the DVD. In fact, in the actual clinical case on which that scenario was based, the patient did not die, although her recovery was quite slow. Her son—as portrayed by the actor in the scenario—was angry about the error and was even more upset when his mother's death was discussed as a possibility, but in the end he said that he was glad that the discussion had been so open.

Here is a "crossroads" to show you some of the options available in the situation in which the relative is asking for reassurance that the patient is not going to die.

➤ *Situation:*

The patient is a woman in her mid-80s who was erroneously given an excess dose of Adriamycin in her chemotherapy. She has just been admitted with septicemia and agranulocytosis. Her current clinical state is grave.

> *The Relative Says:*
> "She's not going to die of this, is she?"
> *You Can Choose From:*
> —*Direct or Factual Response*
>   "No, no."
> —*Escalationary or Judgmental Response*
>   "Of course not!"
> —*Open Question*
>   "What had you been thinking about that?"
> —*Empathic Response*
>   "I realize this is a worrying time for everyone and hard for you. We've started the antibiotics and the support treatments, and while it is possible that she might die, we think that's not very likely—but we'll have a much better idea by the end of today. Can we talk to each other then, and I'll have a better idea of how she's doing and what the future holds?"

Always respond immediately to any emotions expressed by the patient or relative.

See the next section, E: Emotions.

E: *Emotions*

As with all difficult conversations, much depends on your acknowledging the emotions experienced by the other person. Particularly in the context of error disclosure, emotions are likely to be running high. This intensity makes it even more important to acknowledge them. It could even be said that some litigation cases are prompted partly by families' frustration in not feeling that they have been heard—which, as I've said repeatedly, is a result of their feelings of not being acknowledged.

Because you may be reading this section of the book without having read the previous sections, I'm going to repeat the text about the empathic response here, to save your having to flip back and forth. After all, disclosing error is stressful enough; you don't need the added problem of trying to navigate your way through a strategic plan scattered in various places through a book.

The empathic response consists of three steps.

STEP 1: IDENTIFY ONE OF THE EMOTIONS

Most of us experience a mixture of several emotions at the same time. For example, on hearing a piece of bad news, we may feel some fear, some anger, and some disappointment, and we might also have difficulty comprehending it (disbelief) or even want to shut out the news (denial). All of those emotions might coexist behind a shocked "Oh, no!"

So when the patient shows an emotional response (such as "Oh, no!"), you simply need to decide on *one* of the emotions that you can see. (And the fact that you can see the emotional expression clearly shows that it is a "big" experience, something the patient feels intensely and deeply.)

Having fixed on one of the emotions in the mixture, name it (in your own mind). Say to yourself, "This patient is clearly shocked," or "He's angry now," or "She's having difficulty believing what I just said." Don't be afraid of using words with wide, all-inclusive meanings, such as *shock* or *distress* or *upset* and so on.

STEP 2: IDENTIFY THE CAUSE OF THE EMOTION

Usually the cause of the emotion is the piece of news that you have just given or the topic that one of you has just raised. That is all you need. You don't need to perform some miracle of psychoanalysis ("This man is upset because he now sees his career and relationships as total failures and is doubtful that he can recreate his lost youth"). All you need do in step 2 is to pinpoint the immediate cause of the emotional reaction; often it will be something that you have just said.

STEP 3: RESPOND IN A WAY THAT SHOWS YOU HAVE MADE THE CONNECTION BETWEEN STEPS 1 AND 2

Tell the patient that you have observed his or her feelings and that you are aware of what evoked that emotion. Empathic responses (and there are hundreds, of course!) are usually in the form of "Clearly, that's a major shock," or "You are obviously upset by this," or "I realize that this is awful for you," or "This is difficult to take in, isn't it?"

When you respond to a patient's feelings with an empathic response, you achieve three objectives simultaneously:

1. *You legitimize that person's feelings.* You are telling the patient that the emotion he or she is experiencing *is* an understandable response to the situation. In doing that, you are showing that you are not making a judgment about the emotion.

2. *You are telling the person that it is permissible to discuss those feelings.* You are demonstrating that feelings are legitimate items on the agenda between the two of you. In the words of the cliché, "We can talk about this."

3. *You change the subject.* For that moment, you are not talking about the infarct or the hypertension or the bowel cancer; you are talking about how the person *feels* at this moment in response to that information.

In other words, you are showing the patient that you have noted his or her feelings, however briefly, and are including those emotions as part of your overall approach to the clinical situation.

The empathic response, by simply identifying the emotion that is there, is nonjudgmental. When you make an empathic response, you are not making a judgment about whether the emotion is appropriate (in your view) or in proportion (in your view) to the import of the news. You are simply stating that you have seen that the patient is experiencing it.

Of all the things you can do in discussing a medical error, framing empathic responses is the most valuable—provided, of course, that it is followed with an appropriate strategy addressing both the medical condition of the patient and communication with the relatives.

S: Strategy and Summary

The Front-Burner Strategy: Early Follow-up

In disclosing an error, the plan of management—the strategy—is even more important than it is in everyday medical practice.

It is vital that the other person realize that you are taking the situation seriously, and you can demonstrate that by the kind of plan you make for dealing with the situation.

There are two useful guidelines that I find helpful in this situation:

1. MAKE ARRANGEMENTS FOR EARLY AND PROMPT CONTACT

You can create some goodwill by showing the other person that this case is on the "front burner." Often you will find it useful to make contact with each other at the end of the day or even in a couple of hours' time. Always ask the person if he or she would like *you* to call (at a time when you can reliably do that—e.g., the end of the clinic or OR time). I realize that this is not the customary way of doing things, but the patient is likely to realize that fact, too, and will therefore appreciate that this situation is being given your priority attention.

2. GIVE A PHONE NUMBER FOR CONTACT

When a medical error has occurred, I would recommend giving the relative or patient your office number or even your cell number for contact—with specific instructions as to how you can be contacted. Most people at these moments have a fear of being abandoned ("The system has let me down once, it could happen again"), and by simply scribbling your name and number on a scrap of paper and giving it to the person, you are showing that you are part of the solution.

Again—and I know this sounds trivial—let me emphasize that, at times of major stress, the relative or patient is usually anxious about slipping through the cracks and will welcome a clear line of communication.

Summary and Follow-up

At times of uncertainty like this, you should close the interview with a clear brief summary of the situation (as I've said before, this requires a fair amount of mental effort, but it is worth it). Then close with reiterating that the next contact will be soon.

Shaking hands at the end of the interview is helpful, even if the other person is at first somewhat diffident or reluctant. If you shake hands, it changes the relationship slightly; it is more difficult for the relative to maintain anger or opposition to you once you have parted after a handshake.

Of course, disclosure of a medical error is difficult and often provokes anger and/or antagonism.

It is worthwhile your viewing scenario 2 on the DVD. It is also worthwhile visiting the Web site www.sorryworks.net, which has a great deal of relevant material and sources of further information.

In that situation (based on a clinical incident in my own practice), the patient, Mrs. Grant, received the wrong dose of a chemotherapy agent and developed febrile neutropenia. Her son was appropriately angry, and the interview with him illustrates the points that have been mentioned above.

3.5. Other CONES Situations: Bereavement, Sudden Deterioration, Adverse Effects

Bereavement

Informing a relative of the death of a patient is never easy, and it is much harder if the death has been unexpected and sudden. For that reason, it is worthwhile looking at scenario 3 on the accompanying DVD. It illustrates how one might talk to the wife of a young man, with no known history of heart disease, who has just died of an MI during a family picnic.

As you will see, giving the news of bereavement clearly requires a CONES type of approach.

Using a narrative approach, while you are explaining the series of events, you are also listening for two important factors:

1. THE RELATIVE'S UNDERSTANDING OF THE SITUATION AS IT DEVELOPED

As you describe the events, make an effort to see if the relative understands their significance. Check questions, such as "Am I making sense?" or "Do you follow me?" are useful for this purpose.

If the relative indicates that he or she has no idea what the situation is, then it is worthwhile your taking a moment to find out what the person has been told so far. Generally speaking, it is better to ask what the person knows than to make an assumption and later find out you were wrong.

2. THE QUESTION "HAS HE DIED?"

It happens often that as you are progressing along the narrative (the N of CONES), the relative will suddenly say something like, "Oh, my god, he's dead, isn't he?"

This is not always a straightforward matter. But generally, it is almost always better to respond to that vital question straightaway. Any attempt to delay or avoid answering it immediately will be perceived as evasive and disingenuous. However, the way in which you answer that question can help you. The exact words are not crucial. When a relative asks, "Has he died?" any answer that you give apart from "No" will be perceived immediately as "Yes." Hence, you answer with phrases such as "I'm sorry to say that he has died," or "Unfortunately, he is dead," or "We couldn't get the heart restarted, so, yes, I'm sorry to say that he is dead." The point is that when that question is asked, if your first word is not a clear "No," the relative will immediately begin to understand the true situation, that the patient has died.

Although this is very much a matter of personal style, I strongly recommend that you use the words *dead* or *has died* and not euphemisms such as *passed on* or *passed away*. Rarely, such words and euphemisms can be misunderstood (with awkward consequences). This is one of the few moments when the exact words do matter.

3. YOUR OWN EMOTIONS

I am often asked whether it is wrong if you show your own sadness (if that is what you happen to feel) when breaking the bad news of bereavement. The short answer is "No, it is not wrong." In fact, it may be helpful. Some studies carried out in an ER showed that parents of young adults killed in motor vehicle accidents appreciated that the doctor informing them clearly felt sad about the deaths.

It so happens that I have interviewed several widows, some of whom said that their doctors appeared to be somewhat cold and insensitive when telling them of their husbands' death. I have met two or three of those doctors since then, and I can say that those physicians were *not* cold or insensitive. They themselves told me that they had felt that the patient's death was very sad but had had no idea how best to convey the news to the widow.

That is why the empathic response is so valuable. It literally gives you a clue as to what to say—and how to acknowledge the emotion present in the room—when at first you feel that you have no idea what to say.

Using the CONES approach helps you to share news of a bereavement, even though the news is not what anybody wants to hear. When you respond with effective empathic responses to the feelings of the relative, you can be a supportive messenger despite the impact of the message.

Sudden Deterioration

It is reasonable to think of a sudden deterioration in the patient's condition in a way similar to how we think of a patient's death. If the deterioration is significant, then it may help a great deal to inform the relative of that.

The criterion I usually use is to ask myself: "Has this patient's condition changed so much that the spouse would have a shock seeing him today compared with yesterday?" If the answer is *yes*, then it is worthwhile to call the relative. This issue is not of major importance, but if the patient's condition does deteriorate in a major way (particularly in the context of, say, an ICU) and particularly if it was not expected that the patient's condition would deteriorate, then a preemptive conversation in the CONES format may be helpful.

Adverse Effects

What I have been discussing above is also relevant to an adverse effect—even if such a possibility was discussed before starting the treatment. Again, this is not a crucial issue. Furthermore, it is not a medicolegal issue. Although a lot of us may fear that by making contact concerning an adverse event we are taking personal responsibility for it, in fact, the opposite is true. When you make the first contact, you are more likely to be perceived as an observant and helpful physician, as opposed to being blamed as the cause of the problem.

3.6. Summary: Reducing Unease

The CONES approach is not magic!

The strategy set out in CONES offers a way of dealing with an unpleasant situation and may offer you an option at a time when you cannot think of what to do or say. In these difficult circumstances, I make a habit of taking a deep breath and then exhaling slowly when I have my hand on the doorknob before I go into the room, and I repeat the word CONES to myself. At the very least, it offers me a plan.

The HARD Protocol for Resolving Conflict

		Topics covered in this chapter
H	**Hi**gh emotions? **Hi**gh stakes? **H**urried? **H**arried? **H**assled?	Recognize the red flag / danger signals.
A	**A**cknowledge	Acknowledge the situation first to yourself, then verbally to the patient.
R	**R**ules	Overtly state the "rules" or acceptable limits or boundaries of discussion.
D	**D**e-escalate	Once you realize that it may escalate, take steps that de-escalate the interaction.

CHAPTER FOUR

Managing Conflict and Escalation

The HARD Protocol

....

Some solutions that don't make the problems worse

4.1. The Nature of Escalation

....

The one thing that you need to do as a conflict arises is to organize your thoughts. Unfortunately, that ability is often the first casualty of the conflict. The ultimate causes of this problem are now being identified by research in neuroscience. Briefly, a large amount of research data shows that the rage that most of us feel in a conflict has its origins in the activation of the limbic system. To summarize a complex topic, the limbic system is the network of brain centers that includes the amygdaloid nuclei and is partially inhibited and controlled by input from the orbitofrontal cortex. The limbic system is powerful and is activated readily—more rapidly than the neocortex. In fact, it seems likely that the cognitive centers in the cortex lag behind the limbic system by about six seconds. For this reason, we all seem to have difficulty thinking carefully and rationally (cortically, in fact) when in the grip of a limbic rage. To behave rationally (as opposed to emotionally), you need to try to delay your (limbic) urge to react by about six seconds. So, when your grandparents told you to control your temper by "counting to ten," they were right, and in fact their maxim gives you a margin of an extra four seconds to make sure your cortex catches up with and then outpaces your limbic system.

This is how the HARD strategy can help you. If you can make it work, it will help you delay your "limbic rage" by a few seconds and control the urges that would otherwise escalate the conflict.

The HARD strategy has only four simple steps—and you need something that simple. Anything more complex is likely to be swept out of your mind in the tidal wave of escalation. (Please forgive any dramatic language, but it's important that you find this strategy easy to remember at bad times!)

4.2. The HARD Strategy for Attempting to Influence Your Own Feelings

H: *High emotions? High Stakes? Hurried? Harried? Hassled?*

Recognize the red flag

Things are most likely to go wrong when one (or all) of the "five Hs" are involved. When the patient—or you—is feeling angry or upset or is experiencing some other intense emotion, when the medical outcome includes major consequences, when you (or the patient) are in a rush, and/or when there is pressure from outside sources (e.g., many patients to see, calls waiting, visits to organize, etc.)—when any or all of these are going on, the interaction between you and your patient is going to get more difficult.

The first step in disentangling this knot is to recognize the warning signs of its approach. Perhaps the easiest way of achieving that is to learn to recognize your own somatic signs of stress. If you can become aware of your own pulse rate rising or that peculiar whooshing sound in your ears or that churning feeling in your stomach (which is the most reliable indicator in my case) or a strong feeling of "I really dislike this"—if you can learn to recognize any of those as signs of approaching conflict—then you are already on the way to calming the situation.

It is a matter of training yourself to listen to your own internal somatic signs and recognize them as warning signals of an approaching conflict.

A: *Acknowledge*

Tell yourself—and perhaps the other person—that this is getting difficult.

The purpose of recognizing the warning signs of approaching conflict is to acknowledge that fact to yourself—and perhaps to the other person.

If you can manage to do this, you will be on the way to giving your cognitive centers the six seconds that they need to catch up with your limbic system.

Having detected the early somatic warning signs, make a conscious effort to acknowledge them to yourself. It is worth saying to yourself, "I'm feeling tense—this is going to be difficult" or something similar.

At that point you may be able to verbalize the same acknowledgment to the other person. For example, you may be able to say something as brief as, "This is a difficult situation for both of us here." Whether or not you can say that does depend on your own personal style, on your expertise and experience, and on the nature of the relationship and atmosphere that exists between you and the other party. But it is a technique that is worth considering, and once you have used it and seen the benefit it produces, you will feel more comfortable about using it next time.

As is always the case—and a constant theme throughout this book—acknowledgment always makes things better and reduces tension rather than increasing it.

R: Rules

Set out the rules and boundaries as calmly and coolly as you can.
One of the most hazardous assumptions we can make is assuming that all parties in a conflict share the same assumptions!

In handling a conflict, try to set out the rules or boundaries as calmly as you can. Those boundaries or rules or frontiers need to be explained as clearly as you can manage because many conflicts are either initiated or perpetuated by the parties having different (and unspoken) assumptions.

Try to explain what is acceptable and what is unacceptable, and try to do that in as objective and unemotional tone as you can manage. (Merely making the attempt to talk unemotionally will help you achieve that—it will be perceived as your making an effort.)

It is worth saying, "Look, we do have to be reasonable to each other: it's not going to work if you simply insist on getting the treatment a week early," or something similar. When you define the rules or boundaries as objectively as you can manage, you are partially stopping that matter from being simply a personal (and therefore arbitrary) issue between the two of you.

D: De-escalate

Now you can begin to sort this out!
A conflict escalates when both parties feel that they "have no choice" and that there is no alternative open to them other than imposing their will on the other person.

De-escalation is all about finding a compromise, a middle road that is not in its entirety what either party wanted, but is workable and to some extent acceptable. If you want the other party to accept a compromise, you have to be prepared mentally to accept a compromise yourself.

Of course, there are issues that cannot be compromised. If a patient with hypertension is refusing to take the medication, the medical aspects are simple: the blood pressure will not decrease without treatment. That part of the debate is clear, and you can say that (as unemotionally as you can). The important thing is to de-escalate that area of debate by exploring possible paths that are acceptable. To do that you need to find out what is stopping the patient from taking the treatment (it may be a fear of side effects affecting sexual performance, for example) and then propose a de-escalating way forward (for example, trying the treatment for two weeks and changing it if there are side effects).

A compromise is not a matter of blurring or denying the facts. It is a matter of acknowledging the other person's particular set of views and trying to come to an agreement. In the end it achieves results that would not otherwise happen; in the example above, if the de-escalation works, the patient will end up with a lower diastolic. If, on the other hand, the physician had "stuck to his guns," the patient would have taken no treatment and might have had a stroke.

4.3. Summary: Why Little Tricks Have Big Effects

The four steps of HARD do at least offer you the chance of limiting and controlling a dispute before it spreads and becomes generalized. It is easy and common for us to get increasingly infuriated with everything about the other party (a process often called "monstrifying"), and if you can manage to go through the HARD process, there is a good chance that you will often avoid that type of all-out disagreement.

Neuroscience is basically telling us that the design and function of the brain is suboptimal from this point of view. So the HARD strategy can be thought of as a way of partially compensating for a design flaw.

The SAFER Protocol for Giving Information

		Topics covered in this chapter
S	**S**etting and **S**tarting	Setting, greeting, engaging
A	**A**genda	The agenda should be the first item on the agenda.
F	**F**acts	As you give the facts, respond straightaway to emotions and questions.
E	**E**nquiries and **E**motions	The "e" goes on at the same time as the "f."
R	**R**einforcers and **w**rap-up	Reminders (or aides-mémoire) can be jotted notes, brochures, an audiotape (patient's or yours), or a friend or relative.

CHAPTER FIVE

Giving Information Effectively

The SAFER Protocol

···

How to make giving information truly interactive

5.1. The Task of Giving Information

···

It has to be said that often the activity of giving information seems a bit like a chore.

Much of the time, we would prefer it if the patient had obtained a reasonable amount of background information—not too much!—and had a basic understanding of the area, so that we could easily and simply highlight the particular aspects that apply in this case.

Life isn't usually like that.

Furthermore, once we have given all the relevant information to several patients, it is difficult to stop its becoming a bit like a prerecorded message with an unvarying script. As one of my patients said, some of us do have a tendency to slip into telemarketer mode.

In practice, we often have to spend a fair amount of time giving information to our patients. The important thing to realize at the outset is that the *way* you explain things—about the condition, the form of treatment, the side effects, and so on—may have a major effect on the patient's *compliance* and on his or her ability to cope with side effects and other problems as time goes on.

In other words, the time spent on this activity of information giving is a good investment for the future. It is worth expending some effort in optimizing it, because this will affect how the patient perceives—and copes with—whatever occurs later.

Throughout this whole process, keep in mind that there are two areas that may or may not overlap—first, there are the *medical facts* of the condition and its treatment, and second, there are the *issues* that cause the patient great concern which *may or may not* have significance in terms of *health or survival*. For example, you may be discussing the need for a colectomy for, say, long-standing colitis with a high risk of carcinoma. To you, this is a necessary and life-saving intervention. However, the patient may be deeply concerned about the social and sexual sequelae. The patient's concerns are not contradictory to the medical necessity, but they do need to be acknowledged in the discussion (a crucial part of the SAFER protocol).

Apart from the message itself, there are many other aspects that may cause dissatisfaction. A lot of patients say that they feel almost as if they are getting a prefabricated message that tends to sound a bit like a "party line"—an official and dogmatic statement emanating from some medical authority or other.

In essence, this type of dissatisfaction means the patients feel that we seem to be ignoring them as persons (which often means that their emotions have not been acknowledged), and we seem to be "brushing off" concerns that they regarded as important.

For that reason, as you are about to see, the E (emotions and enquiries) and the R (reinforcers) of the SAFER approach help the patient realize that the process is indeed individualized and personal.

5.2. The SAFER Protocol

The essence of personalizing the delivery of information is to acknowledge this particular patient's issues, and that does not mean that you necessarily have to spend a great deal of time doing so. Effective communication is not related to the time spent on it.[1]

S: Setting and Starting

As with all important discussions, get the nonverbal context or setting of the interview right. To save your having to flip back and forth in the book, table 5.1 lists the basic tips that you have encountered in the S (Setting) of SPIKES, the C (Context) of CONES, etc.

Let me say again that when you start the interview well, it helps the situation. It helps you because you are exercising control over some of the

TABLE 5.1   *A Few Basic Tips*

Technique	Central Feature	Notes
Greeting	Use the person's name.	A simple way of establishing the "person" as well as the "problem"
Introduce yourself	Briefly say who you are and what you do.	Merely courteous
Shake hands	Make actual contact.	Don't do that if you have a cold.
Sit down!	Bring your eyes to the same level as the other person's.	Essential
Don't be too far away	Have less than four feet of space between you.	The optimal distance varies with gender and culture, but three feet is rarely wrong.
Adopt a neutral body posture	Look relaxed, or at least not too anxious or irritated.	Even if you don't feel relaxed (and most of us don't at these times), try to adopt the neutral body posture and look relaxed.
Lean forward	Don't sit back all the way against the chair.	Studies show that patients recognize this as a sign of being interested in them.
Be ready to smile	Smiling may not be your usual "thing," but it helps if you can manage it.	If you do smile, try to "smile with your whole face."
Switch on your listening skills	Silence and repetition	Consciously maintain silence as the patient starts talking. Then in your first sentence of response use a word or phrase from the patient's last sentence.

aspects of the interview, and it also helps the patient because you look a bit more comfortable, confident, and in control, and that equates in the patient's mind with increased competence. For that reason, it is worth making a little extra effort to start the interaction off well.

A: Agenda

As the ancient academic adage goes, "Tell them what you're going to tell them, *then* tell them, *then* tell them what you've told them." That is a good guideline for academic teaching, and it's useful in clinical practice, too. Our patients and their accompanying friends are usually fairly anxious, even if, from the medical point of view, you think of the problem as comparatively minor. Somehow, when it's a matter of health and life, the benefits and the risks and the potential consequences all seem to a bit larger than life, and it's difficult for the patient to get a sense of perspective on what you are saying or even to take it in.

This means that it is worth your taking a few seconds thought and setting an agenda so that the patient has some idea of what is coming up. I mean "a few seconds" literally; this is not intended to be a major, detailed, and arduous task. It is just a matter of saying the main topic or topics that you are going to cover. It can be as brief as, "So I'll go ahead and explain what the chemotherapy is like, and how it's given and so on. OK?"

That step in itself seems to make the patient (and the friend or relative) feel a bit more "in the loop." Simply stating the agenda in a few words seems to make people feel more included and acknowledged.

F: Facts

Then explain the main facts.

As I have said before, in the discussing of bad news, it does require a bit of effort to translate your technical jargon—the Medspeak, as it were—into plain language, but it makes all the difference. Naturally, our patients vary in their vocabularies (and in their first languages), so you will be adjusting and finding the level of comprehensibility as you go along. It is worth noting that one cause of patient dissatisfaction with our explaining the facts is the use of words that the patient simply doesn't understand. If you ignore their bafflement and barrel on anyway, the patient will feel deskilled, marginalized, and somewhat belittled. So use plain language and adjust the level to suit this particular patient.

I am strongly in favor of creating—and then giving to the patient—a brief scribbled aide-mémoire. This can be quick and simple. I find that jotting a few words on a scrap of paper is enough. Something memorable seems to happen when you scribble the main headings (two or three words) and one or two words about each point. Perhaps the act of creating the note in front of the patient triggers what is called *contextual learning*. This term refers to the fact that it is easier to memorize information when there is an additional cue in the background (for example, a certain piece of music playing or a certain color of lighting). There is some evidence that people who learn the information while exposed to that cue subsequently have better recall when that cue is reintroduced during the testing period (for example, the same piece of music is played in the background or the same light color is used). I don't know whether or not those scribbled notes act as a trigger for contextual learning, but they do seem to work.

Many physicians nowadays have their own two-part notes printed with the basic headings (e.g., stage of breast cancer, insulin requirements, triggers of asthma, or whatever), which they fill in with the relevant details in front of the patient. They give one copy to the patient, and the other is filed in the chart and is a reminder of the plan of treatment as well as of what information has been shared with the patient.

From what I have seen and heard (from the patients as well as the physicians), this system of fact giving seems to work well.

E: *Enquiries and Emotions (at the Same Time as the Facts)*

Questions and Enquiries

Answering queries and questions is perhaps the most important part of information giving, and while it need not take a great deal of time, it does make the patient feel (appropriately) that the process is being tailored and individualized.

In my own area, oncology, I regard this as a useful investment of time. It may take four minutes, for example, to answer some of the queries about say adjuvant chemotherapy, but those four minutes will alter the patient's attitude to the treatment over the next, say, eighteen weeks and may raise the patient's threshold for coping with the side effects and ability to complete the full course.

A couple of techniques seem to work well for politicians in public and broadcast interviews which I think can also help us.

Pause and Repeat the Question

The basic guideline here is simple: "When you're thinking, you are allowed to pause and say that you're thinking."

In general terms, in everyday practice there is nothing wrong with taking a moment to think, and the act of repeating the question tells the patient that you are thinking about the specific issue that has just been raised. Politicians and spokespeople from all types of organizations use that technique all the time, and it demonstrably works better than blundering straight in with a response that later may be regretted.

Advocacy

There is an enormous difference between saying, "I don't know," and saying, "I don't know but I'll try to find out." The former carries an implication of finality and also an element of abandonment, whereas the latter states clearly that the issue now involves some form of advocacy on your part. Importantly, if you say that you will try to find out further information, you have to do that. Even sending a message a few days later that you don't yet have the answer is a valuable transaction in your relationship. Another useful hint for busy practitioners: You can ask the patient to call your office if you haven't made contact in the next few days. (We all have "to-do" lists that grow rather than shrink.)

Emotions

As I have mentioned many times in this book so far, as you give new information to the patient, it is essential that you acknowledge and respond to the emotional component of the patient's reactions to that information. The empathic response is the most practical way of doing that, and in case you happen to be reading this section without having read the preceding parts, I shall once again reproduce the text describing it, so that you don't have to flip back and forth (an activity that often goes wrong under the duress of a clinic or office session).

The empathic response consists of three steps.

STEP 1: IDENTIFY ONE OF THE EMOTIONS

Most of us experience a mixture of several emotions at the same time. For example, on hearing a piece of bad news, we may feel some fear, some anger, and some disappointment, and we might also have difficulty comprehending it (disbelief) or even want to shut out the news (denial). All of those emotions might coexist behind a shocked "Oh, no!"

So when the patient shows an emotional response (such as "Oh, no!"), you simply need to decide on *one* of the emotions that you can see. (And the fact that you can see the emotional expression clearly shows that it is a "big" experience, something the patient feels intensely and deeply.)

Having fixed on one of the emotions in the mixture, name it (in your own mind). Say to yourself, "This patient is clearly shocked," or "He's angry now," or "She's having difficulty believing what I just said." Don't be afraid of using words with wide, all-inclusive meanings, such as *shock* or *distress* or *upset* and so on.

STEP 2: IDENTIFY THE CAUSE OF THE EMOTION

Usually the cause of the emotion is the piece of news that you have just given or the topic that one of you has just raised. That is all you need. You don't need to perform some miracle of psychoanalysis ("This man is upset because he now sees his career and relationships as total failures and is doubtful that he can recreate his lost youth"). All you need do in step 2 is to pinpoint the immediate cause of the emotional reaction; often it will be something that you have just said.

STEP 3: RESPOND IN A WAY THAT SHOWS YOU HAVE MADE THE CONNECTION BETWEEN STEPS 1 AND 2

Tell the patient that you have observed his or her feelings and that you are aware of what evoked that emotion. Empathic responses (and there are hundreds, of course!) are usually in the form of "Clearly, that's a major shock," or "You are obviously upset by this," or "I realize that this is awful for you," or "This is difficult to take in, isn't it?"

When you respond to a patient's feelings with an empathic response, you achieve three objectives simultaneously:

1. *You legitimize that person's feelings.* You are telling the patient that the emotion he or she is experiencing *is* an understandable response to the situation. In doing that, you are showing that you are not making a judgment about the emotion.

2. *You are telling the person that it is permissible to discuss those feelings.* You are demonstrating that feelings are legitimate items on the agenda between the two of you. In the words of the cliché: "We can talk about this."

3. *You change the subject.* For that moment, you are not talking about the infarct or the hypertension or the bowel cancer; you are

talking about how the person *feels* at this moment in response to that information.

In other words, you are showing the patient that you have noted his or her feelings, however briefly, and are including those emotions as part of your overall approach to the clinical situation.

R: Reinforcers and Wrap-up

"Never mind the medium; the message is the message."

There isn't any incontrovertible evidence that one method of reinforcing the information is consistently better than all the others.

Reminders and reinforcers consist of anything—notes, brochures, tapes, hints, phone numbers, etc.—that you give to the patient at the end of the meeting to provide further information as well as to help him or her recall what you have discussed and methods of contact and follow-up.

Some form of written or printed material seems to be helpful. As I've just said, I recommend the scribbled notes you made during the explanation and/or any printed material (for instance pharmacy tear-off sheets about the drugs to be used, which you can tell the patients they will get from the pharmacy). Possibly the scribbled notes facilitate a form of contextual learning as I mentioned above, and when the patient gets home the written aid may bring back memories of much of the interview.

There have been some studies about the use of audio recordings (made either by physicians or patients) during the interview. The studies suggest that they are helpful, but I must admit that I find there is a somewhat stultifying effect of having a recorder running during the discussions. Somehow all parties are more inclined to talk more formally and legalistically.

Of course, Web sites and chat rooms are often useful—again, a brochure or booklet with the URL of a few recommended Web sites is helpful.

You're Allowed to Call "Time"

Time management is rarely easy for us in clinical medicine, but, of course, it is a standard and crucial part of the practice of psychiatry, psychotherapy, and other counseling disciplines. The basic message is that we are allowed to close the current interview provided that (1) the biggest and most significant topics have been raised and discussed, (2) closing the interview is discussed a few minutes before it occurs (not suddenly—by walking out, for example!), (3) the interview is ended in a calm and unemotional manner, and (4) if necessary, you either make an appointment for the next visit or tell the patient how that appointment will be arranged.

It is highly unlikely that you will be able to discuss every facet and feature of all the patient's problems and concerns (see figure in introduction, p. 5) and with a few patients (such as those who have borderline personality disorder[2]) it may not be possible, no matter how much time is allocated.

The secret in calling "time" is to state the time limits as calmly and unhurriedly as possible, with as little emotion as you can, and to make a genuine offer to have a further interview if required or possible. You are allowed to say things such as, "So we won't make a further appointment, but your family doctor can let me know if there's a new problem in the future."

5.3. Summary: Making the Routine Fresh

The secret of a successful information-giving interview is to make it seem fresh and memorable to the patient—no matter how often you have covered the ground with other patients. The best way to do that is to respond to the patient's expressed emotions and personal questions. If you do this and if you are reasonably good at closing the interview when time runs out, then you will not feel oppressed by these interviews (and neither will your patients!).

The CONERS Protocol for Requesting Autopsy or Organ Donation

		Topics covered in this chapter
C	**C**ontext	Setting, greeting, engaging
O	**O**pening remark	Include "sorry" for bereavement.
N	**N**arrative	Explain (at length) the chronology of events, including the uncertainties.
E	**E**motions	Respond to (acknowledge) all emotions and questions.
R	**R**equest	Only *after* that, make request for organ donation or autopsy.
S	**S**trategy and **S**ummary	Explain details of how relative will be told. Give contact numbers.

CHAPTER SIX

Some Particularly Difficult Conversations

Good approaches at bad times

6.1. Requests for Autopsy or for Organ Donation

Discussions about autopsies and organ donation are never easy. By their very nature, these conversations are held at times of high emotion and distress, times at which most people simply don't want to be bothered with discussions and decisions about other matters. Therefore, the key to tackling these subjects successfully is to realize that there is a clear delineation between the human tragedy involved, on the one hand, and the request for autopsy or organ donation, on the other.

For that reason, I find that it works best if you address the human part of the conversation first (i.e., the death, the bereavement, and the emotions created thereby) and *then* come to the request. For that reason, I would recommend that you use the CONES approach to holding a dialogue about the death, modified by adding the request *after* you have acknowledged the emotions. We can call this modification of the CONES strategy the CONERS approach.

Once again, some of this material will be familiar to you if you have read other parts of this book. I apologize for the duplication, but I want the book to be helpful for any reader who just grabs it for these particular tasks. These situations are ones in which the need to flip backward and forward in a book is frustrating—as it is even at the best of times, but much more so if there are anxious and distressed relatives nearby!

C: Context

In the difficult situation of needing to have a discussion after a death, fixing the physical *context* of the interview, the greeting, and *opening remark* all *occur at the same time,* so there is not any separation in time between the C (context) and the O (opening remark). I am separating them here simply so that I can say a few things about each of them, but in clinical practice they occur simultaneously.

The most important thing about the context—the physical setting of the interview—is to create a feeling of privacy. Even if you have no choice but to hold the discussion in a waiting room or somewhere a bit more public, you can still create a feeling (albeit illusory) of privacy if you come close to the other person—say, with two or three feet of space between you—and get your eyes on the same level as hers or his.

As you come in, shake hands with the person and, at the same time, if you haven't met the person before, say who you are and what you do. Then immediately go straight on to the opening remark.

O: Opening

After a death, if the relative knows that the patient has died, it is totally reasonable to start with an acknowledgement of the bereavement as your first words. Most physicians do that, and they express their condolences at the start, while they are shaking hands with the relative.

This seems sensible and fits in with accepted social norms. I think it is worth being specific and saying something like, "I am so sorry about your husband's death." Many people say, "I am sorry for your loss," which seems to work well for them. Others will just say, "Sorry," which in this context is also fine.

Circumstances vary widely, and it may happen that the relatives know a lot about what went on, but it is worth finding out if there are any questions. I often say something like, "You may know a lot about what happened, but would you like me to give you a brief summary of it so you can ask any questions that you want to?" This approach basically establishes whether or not the relative has some major unanswered questions and/or wants to hear a summary of the situation that reinforces what they have already been told or have understood.

The important thing is that after the Opening Remark you will move on to the descriptive Narrative, while simultaneously dealing with Emotions and Enquiries.

N: Narrative

The main value of giving a brief overview of the events is to give the relatives some time to gather their own thoughts *and*—most important—to have the opportunity to (1) ask any unanswered questions, and (2) to express their emotions. In the other words, a main function of the narrative is to give a structure in which emotions can be expressed by the relatives and acknowledged by you.

For that reason, your narrative can be brief and can contain wish statements. You might say something like "After a major stroke such as your husband had, we were hoping for some degree of recovery—as sometimes happens. Sadly, that didn't happen, though we all wish it had." Then listen for the two types of response that I have just mentioned: (1) unanswered questions and (2) emotional components.

In discussing the death of the patient, it is essential that you answer the question, "Has he died?" *immediately* and *empathically*.

This is not a question to which the answer can be postponed. Furthermore, at this crucial juncture in the interview, any answer other than "no" will be construed as "yes." Hence, if you begin your reply with "I'm very sorry to tell you that sadly your husband . . ." by the time you have completed the first four or five words, the relative will have realized that the patient has in fact died. Of course the news may be devastating, but if you follow the guidelines in the last few paragraphs, you will be perceived as a supportive messenger bearing an unpleasant message.

E: Emotions and Enquiries

As with all difficult conversations, much depends on your acknowledging the emotions experienced by the other person. Particularly in the context of a recent death, emotions are likely to be running high. This makes it even more important to acknowledge them.

Because you may be reading this section of the book without having read the previous sections, I'm going to repeat the text about the empathic response here, to save your having to flip back and forth. After all, requests for autopsy or for organ donation are stressful enough; you don't need the added problem of trying to navigate your way through a strategic plan scattered in various places through a book.

The empathic response consists of three steps.

STEP 1: IDENTIFY ONE OF THE EMOTIONS

Most of us experience a mixture of several emotions at the same time. For example, on hearing a piece of bad news, we may feel some fear, some anger, and some disappointment, and we might also have difficulty comprehending it (disbelief) or even want to shut out the news (denial). All of those emotions might coexist behind a shocked "Oh, no!"

So when the patient shows an emotional response (such as "Oh, no!"), you simply need to decide on *one* of the emotions that you can see. (And the fact that you can see the emotional expression clearly shows that it is a "big" experience, something the patient feels intensely and deeply.)

Having fixed on one of the emotions in the mixture, name it (in your own mind). Say to yourself, "This patient is clearly shocked," or "He's angry now," or "She's having difficulty believing what I just said." Don't be afraid of using words with wide, all-inclusive meanings, such as *shock* or *distress* or *upset* and so on.

STEP 2: IDENTIFY THE CAUSE OF THE EMOTION

Usually the cause of the emotion is the piece of news that you have just given or the topic that one of you has just raised. That is all you need. You don't need to perform some miracle of psychoanalysis ("This man is upset because he now sees his career and relationships as total failures and is doubtful that he can recreate his lost youth"). All you need do in step 2 is to pinpoint the immediate cause of the emotional reaction; often it will be something that you have just said.

STEP 3: RESPOND IN A WAY THAT SHOWS YOU HAVE MADE THE CONNECTION BETWEEN STEPS 1 AND 2

Tell the patient that you have observed his or her feelings and that you are aware of what evoked that emotion. Empathic responses (and there are hundreds, of course!) are usually in the form of "Clearly, that's a major shock," or "You are obviously upset by this," or "I realize that this is awful for you," or "This is difficult to take in, isn't it?"

When you respond to a patient's feelings with an empathic response, you achieve three objectives simultaneously:

1. *You legitimize that person's feelings.* You are telling the patient that the emotion he or she is experiencing *is* an understandable response to the situation. In doing that, you are showing that you are not making a judgment about the emotion.

2. *You are telling the person that it is permissible to discuss those feelings.* You are demonstrating that feelings are legitimate items on the agenda between the two of you. In the words of the cliché: "We can talk about this."

3. *You change the subject.* For that moment, you are not talking about the infarct or the hypertension or the bowel cancer; you are talking about how the patient *feels* at this moment in response to that information.

In other words, you are showing the patient that you have noted his or her feelings, however briefly, and are including those emotions as part of your overall approach to the clinical situation.

The empathic response, by simply identifying the emotion that is there, is nonjudgmental. When you make an empathic response, you are not making a judgment on whether the emotion is appropriate (in your view) or in proportion (in your view) to the import of the news. You are simply stating that you have seen that the patient is experiencing emotion.

R: Request

Some relatives have already made up their minds about an autopsy or organ donation, but even if that is the case, you will not have lost any ground by acknowledging their emotions before you make the request. If they haven't made up their minds already, then of course this is the logical point in the discussion to make the request.

As I've said often in this book, it helps to acknowledge verbally anything that tends to affect or inhibit the discussion. The difficulty in introducing what might be an awkward topic is a good example. You will find it helpful to acknowledge that awkwardness.

Examples of phrases you can use to introduce the subject:
- "Now I'm afraid I have to ask you about something that is probably difficult for you."
- "I'd like us to talk about a rather difficult subject."
- "I'd like to ask you about a subject that a lot of people find a bit difficult."
- "Now this is a difficult subject to talk about, but it is important."

The way you phrase the request—as with most of the situations in this book—is not very important. What matters is how you respond to the relative's reaction.

A Request for Autopsy
➤ *Situation:*
The patient has just died in his mid-60s of complications of diabetes. You are asking the widow for permission to perform an autopsy.

The Next of Kin Says:
"No. He's suffered enough."
You Can Choose From:
—*Direct or Factual Response*
   "So you're refusing permission, then."
—*Escalationary or Judgmental Response*
   "It's got absolutely nothing to do with suffering."
—*Open Question*
   "Tell me what you're thinking of."
—*Empathic Response*
   "I understand what you're saying. And a lot of people feel like that. But his suffering is over now. And an autopsy will help us understand more about the details of how the condition behaved."

A Request for Organ Donation
➤ *Situation:*
The patient has just died after a head injury in a vehicle accident. He had a signed organ donation card on him, but hospital regulations make asking permission from the next of kin mandatory.

The Next of Kin Says:
"I'm so upset; I just can't think this through. No. It just doesn't feel right. No."
You Can Choose From:
—*Direct or Factual Response*
   "So you're refusing permission, then."
—*Escalationary Or Judgmental Response*
   "So you're denying a chance at life for someone else?"
—*Open Question*
   "Are you able to tell me what makes you say that?"
—*Empathic Response*
   "I understand what you say when you say it doesn't feel right. Perhaps it never does. But do take some time and think about it again—it would help other people to live."

S: Strategy

There is only one important point about the procedure for both autopsy and organ donation: the administrative steps must be simple and must require no effort from the next of kin. For that reason, it is worth your familiarizing yourself with the process in advance if you don't know it already. It is helpful if you can say something such as, "Fortunately, the process itself is simple—you just go to Office 320 on the third floor and they'll ask you to sign a straightforward form."

6.2. Other Specific Difficult Situations

Transition to Palliative Care

The topic of communication in the context of palliative care merits a full discussion of its own, which is too lengthy (and probably not appropriate) for this book. For that reason, I think it is worthwhile consulting one of the several major textbooks on palliative care, all of which have sections on communication. There are several available as well as the one in which I wrote the section on communication.[1]

Transition to palliative care is such an important topic in all areas of clinical practice, not only in oncology. When the objectives of treatment are moved from the goal of curing or containing the condition to the achievable goals of controlling symptoms, there is always considerable disappointment (on the part of the doctor as well as the patient).

The SPIKES approach is helpful here.

When you know the patient well, you can give a brief overview of recent events and check that the patient has a realistic perception (P) of the current situation. If you do not know the patient well, you can of course ask for his or her perception of the situation ("ask before you tell").

➤ *Situation:*

The patient has non-small-cell lung cancer, which has now progressed on the third line of therapy. There are no further options for treatment of the disease.

> *The Patient Says:*
> "Do you mean I'm going to die of this?"
> *You Can Choose From:*
> —*Direct or Factual Response*
>   "I'm sorry to say that's the way it looks now."
> —*Escalationary or Judgmental Response*
>   "Look, we've done our best. It's not my fault the treatment hasn't worked."
> —*Open Question*
>   "Why don't you tell me what you think?"
> —*Empathic Response*
>   "I know this is hard for you. Why don't you tell me what you think of the situation?"

Conversations about DNR Orders

Conversations about Do Not Resuscitate (DNR) orders have changed over the last few years.

In many institutions, as recently as a decade ago, the decision about a DNR order was regarded as the personal choice of the patient. No matter what the circumstances and even if the possibility of cardiopulmonary resuscitation (CPR) succeeding was zero, the final decision as to whether resuscitation should be attempted was viewed as that of the patient solely.

The conversation about DNR orders was thus regarded as an "informed consent" discussion, in which the patient had to express a wish for a DNR order to be written before it could be written.

In other words, several years ago it might have happened that a patient could be at the end of life with several untreatable conditions (say, for example, a man in his late 70s might have severe emphysema, multi-infarct dementia, diabetes with chronic renal failure, and vascular problems). Yet, even if the patient clearly understood and acknowledged the imminence of his death, *if* he expressed a wish that resuscitation be attempted, he had that right, and a DNR ordered could *not* be written.

This did not make sense to me or seem consistent with the use of CPR as a specific treatment for cardiac arrest rather than as a "treatment for death." To explore this further, I conducted a small survey asking patients who had discussed the issue with their physician and who had acknowledged their own imminent deaths and were already on waiting lists for palliative care institutions (where no CPR facilities are available).[2] I asked the patients whether they would wish us (i.e., the medical team) to attempt to restart their heart if it stopped. (At the time this was the mandatory way of holding a discussion about DNR orders.)

The results were somewhat surprising. One third of those patients—all of whom had already held discussions about dying—nevertheless still wanted CPR when it was offered in the way mandated by our hospital regulations.

For those reasons—as well as several others—many organizations began to reexamine the nature of a DNR conversation and recognized that there was an allure (some called it "the intoxicating effect") of a discussion about a therapy that is known to be futile in those circumstances. In other words, over a period of time it was recognized that discussions about CPR with a dying patient created illusions.

As a result, and after many years of debate and discussion, many institutions all over the world now no longer require (as a mandated obligation on the medical staff) discussion about CPR *specifically* as an intervention, as long as the patient clearly understands that he or she is dying, that death is imminent, and that the entire objective of clinical care is comfort and symptomatic relief.

Hence, the situation in many institutions at present requires the physician and the dying patient to discuss the objectives of treatment and to discuss the implications of palliation being the entire objective of care, with no further prescribed or planned treatment directed against the disease(s).

In those circumstances, as long as the patient clearly understands the prognosis and the imminence of death, the staff are not obliged to discuss CPR specifically.

In other institutions, the rules are different. Some institutions still regard DNR orders as if it were a procedure for which informed consent must be obtained.

So it is important, therefore, that before you have this type of discussion with patients you find out precisely what the regulations in your own hospital or clinic are.

If your institution regulations require you to ask about CPR as an "informed consent" type of discussion, here is how you might use an empathic response to open a discussion, rather than use a direct or an escalation response to solidify a confrontation.

➤ *Situation:*
The patient in his late 70s has multisystem failure with rising creatinine, falling po_2, and congestive cardiac failure unresponsive to inotropes. He has also had several strokes. You are obliged by hospital regulations to ask him about his wishes regarding attempts to restart his heart if it stops.

The Patient Says:
"Oh, sure! Who wouldn't want the chance to get his heart started again?"
You Can Choose From:
—*Direct or Factual Response*
"So you want us to try, even though it won't work and may break a lot of ribs?"
—*Escalationary or Judgmental Response*
"That's not a very intelligent choice, given your situation."
—*Open Question*
"Tell me what's going through your mind."
—*Empathic Response*
"These aren't easy things to talk about, are they? Tell me what you expect from CPR."

"But the Surgeon Said He Got It All"

Many times your patient will tell you something that he or she has been told by another staff member which conflicts with what you have said about the situation or treatment. This is almost always a tricky situation. However, there are three key points in approaching this issue.

1. YOU WEREN'T PRESENT WHEN THE OTHER PERSON GAVE THE INFORMATION

Hence, you are now relying on what the patient recalls and understands about what was said; there is no objective measure that will establish some gold-standard truth. Even if the chart contains a note from the other staff member, the patient may say, "Well, that's not what he actually said" and you are entering a he-said-she-said dispute.

2. HOW DOES THE PATIENT FEEL ABOUT THIS NOW?

This is a situation in which open questions followed by empathic responses to the emotions are valuable. By exploring what the patient now feels about what was said previously and by then acknowledging the emotions, you completely avoid making judgments or taking sides. Often we will be tempted either to act defensively and defend what the other person said or (occasionally) to side with the patient in condemning what he or she understood from what the staff member said. Open questions followed by empathic responses are extremely useful here.

➤ *Situation:*
The patient is a 46-year-old woman who has a small node-positive receptor positive breast cancer. Adjuvant chemotherapy is indicated.

The Patient Says:
"But the surgeon said he got it all!"
You Can Choose From:
—*Direct or Factual Response*
  "It's not possible to 'get it all.' That's why we need to follow up with chemotherapy."
—*Escalationary or Judgmental Response*
  "Well, he was wrong. And he shouldn't have said that."

—Open Question
"Tell me what you understood by that."
—Empathic Response
"You sound disappointed."

3. ALWAYS EMPHASIZE THE BIOLOGY OF THE MEDICAL CONDITION

Another useful hint is to emphasize the behavior—and the unpredict-ability—of the medical condition. (This is particularly true in medical oncology, but it also applies to virtually any discipline.) The truth is that most medical conditions contain some element of unpredictability, and there are often unanswerable questions about whether the treatment plan will work, over what time frame, and with what side effects.

When you underline the best-case and worst-case scenarios in such situations, you are emphasizing your experience or knowledge of the situation and also implying that you have some role in the future care.

6.3. Summary: Listen before You Ask

In this chapter, we've looked at a few difficult situations in which ac-knowledging the other person's emotion is of paramount importance and may play a crucial role in the subsequent discussion of the issue: whether it is organ donation, a request for autopsy, or changing the other person's understanding of the situation. The bottom line is the same one that runs through this whole book: You need to acknowledge strong emotions be-fore any detailed discussion can continue.

The ROSE Protocol for Preparing for a Difficult Conversation

		Topics covered in this chapter
R	**R**ecognize the tough, "high stakes" interviews	Recognize the red flag / danger signals: recurrence, progressive disease, transition to palliative care, medical error.
O	**O**rganize your **o**bjectives	What would you like to happen by the end of this interview? Think through first to yourself, then perhaps express verbally to the patient.
S	**S**trategize	What kind of strategy or approach will help most (e.g., SPIKES, CONES, HARD, SAFER)?
E	**E**xhale	With your hand on the door handle before you go into the room, take a deep breath in and let it out slowly. You're going to do as well as possible!

Putting It All Together and Making a Difference in Communication

These are all tips that you can use.

How you express a thought—and which thought you choose to express—changes the relationship between you and the other person. A great deal of the negative feelings (private and public) created during medical discussions are caused by the physician's not having a plan or approach in mind and being caught off guard, which often triggers defensive and evasive conversation.

The protocols I have discussed so far do at least set out logical and helpful approaches. Simply following these guidelines will greatly change the patient's perception of the outcome. Now let us think about whether we can in some way organize our thoughts before the interview.

Getting Ready: The ROSE Approach to Advance Planning

Sometimes you can partially prepare for a difficult interview.

Perhaps the following observation may seem a bit like a Zen cliché ("Prepare for the things that might catch you unprepared"), but sometimes we can spot potential trouble in advance and partially think through the strategies that might help us in handling it. Of course, it is the totally unexpected situations that are a major cause of difficulty, but sometimes you can see the turbulence approaching, and sometimes you can prepare for it.

The secret is to start by recognizing those clinical situations in which there is likely to be difficulty.

The ROSE checklist is a way of alerting ourselves to an impending problem and thinking about ways we might handle it.

R: Recognize the "High Stakes" Interviews in Advance

Probably you do most of this already. Just before you see the patient, there are common situations that wave a red flag at you and seem to send a warning signal.

Whenever you sense that "red flag" type of interaction coming, *take it seriously* (as the rest of the ROSE checklist will help you to do).

The clinical situations that will probably trigger a red flag are ones such as these:

- An unexpected abnormal test result (particularly if both you and the patient had been expecting a normal result)
- An abnormal result of a screening test
- Adverse reactions to medication
- Significant deterioration in clinical state
- Psychiatric problems including depression, anxiety
- Social and relationship difficulties (e.g., an estranged spouse or a relative who has made a long journey)
- Recurrence of a medical condition (particularly psychiatric) that had seemed to be stable or absent
- Discussion of a medical error

There are, of course, dozens of other categories, but many of them are partially identifiable in advance. For example, in my own area, oncology, some situations are common and are almost always fraught with tension:

- Disease progression after a period of remission or stability
- Transition to palliative care
- Discussions about DNR (Do Not Resuscitate) orders

In oncology, these situations are recognizable and always tough. The peculiar thing is that they don't get easier as we get older, either. All that happens is that as we become more experienced we can see our way through the apparent chaos; we have (a little) more confidence in our ability to handle the situation, because it has happened before. That may be one of the major advantages of recognizing a situation in advance: not only can you reckon up the *size* of the task ahead but also you can *compare* it with other occasions when you've had to handle similar situations.

O: *Organize Your Objectives*

The big practical advantage of organizing your objectives comes when you make it simple.

As you take in the clinical situation, you will probably realize in an instant the difficulty that confronts you and the patient. If the fasting glucose result is high, or the bone scan shows recurrence of the cancer, or the stress test shows ischemic heart disease, you instantly realize the significance of those results.

The secret in maximizing the value of your interaction with the patient —of improving the flow through the middle of the hourglass (if you recall that analogy; see the Introduction)—is to take a couple of seconds to restate your task in your mind. It need be no more than "The cancer has recurred, and I'm going to have to tell her that," or "This heart problem needs to be sorted out, and he was planning on going abroad. I'm going to have to tell him that."

As you organize the objectives of this interview, you can make them as simple and as straightforward as you like. Simply having some plan of what you want to achieve in the interview is a good start.

S: *Strategize*

Having told yourself what you would like to achieve, then spend another two seconds deciding on which approach will help you best. For example, if this patient is new to you and has colorectal cancer, then you might decide that SPIKES is going to be a useful strategy. Or if you have just found out that an error has occurred, then CONES might be your chosen tactic. Whatever it is, just think briefly through the few major points. It's the same as planning a journey. You quickly think, "I get on to the highway, then take that first exit at Rochester, then that road to Broadgate," and so on.

All you need do is to give yourself a simple map. Personally, I repeat the strategy that I'm going to use under my breath a couple of times because it reminds me that I do have some idea of how I'm going to approach the problem.

E: Exhale

Take in a deep breath and let it out slowly.

I know what you're thinking! You're thinking that performing this maneuver is a gimmick or a trick. Well, in a way, you're right. It *is* a trick, but it's a trick that your rational brain plays on your own limbic system (see section 4.1, p. 91). What you do as you take in a breath and then exhale is to stamp your own cognitive control on a situation where the biggest hazard is that the first-placed emotional response (mediated by the limbic system) might cause events to get out of control completely.

Even if it sounds a little gimmicky to you right now as you read this, please try it next time you come to a sticky situation. Once you've seen how it helps, you'll use it the time after that—and it'll be even more helpful. It's like a talisman or a lucky charm. The magic doesn't come from the talisman or the charm at all; it comes from the increased sense of control and competence that the talisman gives you.

Try it. You'll be impressed at your newfound abilities!

As I've said before, the object of the whole exercise is to do what our grandparents told us: when you feel cross, count to ten. The ROSE strategy is no more than a fancy way of counting to ten (probably more like counting to five now that the demands on our time are so intense!) and using those few seconds to make some useful preparations.

In Conclusion

From here on, it's up to you.

The importance of setting all this out in a book (and on DVD) is that you can see various strategies (not scripts) for approaching difficult conversations. I hope that this reassures you that all of us experience difficulty some of the time. As we get older, we continue to feel perplexed and perhaps embarrassed by these situations, but we gradually get better at not showing that. As has been said, "We all still blush, but after a time the blush stays below the clavicles."

Perhaps the greatest difficulty comes when you simply have no idea of how to approach the situation or what to say. I hope this book and the DVD give you a few hints as to how you can start the process with your patient. In fact, the patient will see as positive the mere fact that you want to try to communicate empathically.

Communication is often the only modality immediately available to us. It has a wide therapeutic range (overdose is almost unheard of); it has relatively few side effects and is often given in suboptimal doses. I hope this book has given you some ideas of administration.

Good communication matters, and it is often the main criterion by which our overall performance as health care professionals is judged. When we communicate badly and insensitively, our patients will rarely forgive us, but when we communicate effectively and acknowledge our patients' feelings, they will rarely forget us.

I wish you all the best.

Acknowledgments

··

I have had some wonderful teachers and role models as well as, more recently, some superb collaborators and (forgive the slang) co-conspirators.

In the first group, my mentors and inspirations, I owe a great deal to the late Dr. Eve Wiltshaw, a superb and thoughtful medical oncologist who was also intuitively talented at acknowledging how her patients felt.

With Dr. Peter Maguire I later made my first series of videos on the breaking of bad news, and then after emigrating to Canada, with the help of Dr. Yvonne Kason, wrote *How to Break Bad News*.

Since the mid-1980s, I have been collaborating with Dr. Walter Baile at the M.D. Anderson, and we have produced two sets of CD-ROMs (*A Practical Guide to Communication Skills in Clinical Practice* and *A Practical Guide to Communication Skills in Cancer Care*) as well as a video about the personal burdens of the discipline, entitled *On Being an Oncologist,* presented by the actors William Hurt and Megan Cole. Recently, Walter has designed and set up the I*CARE Web site as part of the M.D. Anderson site, and you can find many of our videotaped scenarios (and much else besides) by going to www.mdanderson.org/icare.

In many respects, this entire book has centered on the importance of acknowledgments in all our communications with each other, so it is perhaps highly appropriate to acknowledge that very fact in the last sentence of it.

Appendix

....

Notes to Accompany the Scenarios on DVD

These notes are a brief guide to the scenarios that you will see on the DVD. It's important to remember that each of them is completely unrehearsed and un-scripted—the actor playing the patient was only briefed on the medical condition and the personality and personal history of the patient she or he portrays. These scenarios show how protocols (SPIKES and CONES) can work in practice, but they are by no means perfect. There may be many things that you think could have been done more effectively and better. That activity—of thinking through how you would have handled the situation—is part of the purpose of using them.

A.1. Recurrence of Bowel Cancer

The Clinical Situation

THE PATIENT

Mrs. Wright had a stage II colorectal carcinoma removed three years ago. Because four lymph nodes were involved, she had adjuvant chemotherapy with 5FU and leucovorin (six courses). She was completely well in follow-up with a normal CEA until about four weeks ago, when she began to feel noticeably more tired than usual and noted a slight and mild ache in her right upper quadrant. The latest CEA had risen to 15. You booked a CT scan to be done in a few days' time, and you repeated the CEA.

THE SETTING

She returns to the clinic to hear the results. The CEA has now risen to 18, and the CT shows six small (1–2 cm) lesions scattered through both lobes of the liver.

Preinterview Plans

Thinking over the situation in the seconds before the interview starts, it is clear that this is going to be a "high stakes" interaction, so the R task of ROSE is to recognize (and give yourself a "heads-up" alert) that this is going to be an important discussion.

In the O for Organize, it is also clear that the bad news about the recurrence has to be given to the patient. So, as regards S for Strategy, the approach that will probably work best is the SPIKES protocol.

Because Mrs. Wright is known to you, the P for Perception can be more a matter of going over the reasons for the CT—a recap of the recent events—rather than a full explanation from square one of the situation. With all that in mind, you take a deep breath in and exhale (the E of ROSE) before starting the discussion.

Points to Watch For

Note that the preceding events are recapitulated, checking that the patient has an accurate perception (the P of SPIKES), and then the physician goes directly on to set out the agenda or the order of events (the I of SPIKES).

What Could Have Been Done Differently?

Would it have been better to launch straight in to the results of the CT? Would it have been (1) possible or (2) desirable to avoid conversation about the future and, for example, the children? At the end of the interview, how do you think Mrs. Wright rated the way she was given the information?

A.2. Disclosing Error

The Clinical Situation

THE PATIENT AND HER SON

Mrs. Grant, an 81-year-old woman, was diagnosed with lymph-node positive breast cancer four weeks ago. It was grade III (undifferentiated) and hormone-receptor negative and *her2* negative. She had no other medical problems and was living independently with a full range of outdoor and indoor daily activities (i.e., ECOG performance status 0).

After discussion with the patient and her son, it was agreed that she should have adjuvant chemotherapy with three courses of 5-fluorouracil, Adriamycin, and cyclophosphamide (FAC), followed by three courses of docetaxel.

She was given the first dose of FAC ten days ago. She tolerated the chemotherapy well, as regards mild nausea and fatigue. Unfortunately, last night she suddenly developed a fever with rigors and felt very ill. She was admitted via the ER and was found to have a WBC of 0.2 with zero neutrophils. She has been started on IV antibiotics and dehydration.

You have reviewed her chart and realize that she inadvertently received too high a dose of Adriamycin—about 175 percent of the correct dose.

Mrs. Grant's son has been asked to meet with you this morning. You have only just discovered the medication error, and he does not yet know of it.

Preinterview Plans

In quickly thinking through the ROSE checklist, obviously this is going to be a difficult interview. The objective will be to inform Mr. Grant of the error, and the best strategy is the CONES approach. You take a deep breath and exhale slowly before Mr. Grant comes in.

Points to Watch For

Mr. Grant is appropriately angry and is clearly angry about the situation and the possibility—even if remote—of his mother's death. Mr. Grant is also clearly a busy and successful man. Plans for follow-up obviously will have to fit in with his schedule.

What Could Have Been Done Differently?

Could anything have been said differently that would have changed Mr. Grant's reactions? What strategy would you suggest for follow-up with Mr. Grant?

A.3. Informing a Relative of the Patient's Death

The Clinical Situation

THE PATIENT

Mr. Lane, a man in his early 40s with no previous history of heart disease, experienced sudden chest pain and collapsed while at a family picnic. He was rushed by ambulance to the ER, where he was found to have had a large MI. During resuscitation, he developed electromechanical dissociation. After many minutes of zero cardiac output, he was declared dead. You now have to tell this to Mrs. Lane, who is waiting in the relatives' room in the ER.

THE RELATIVE

You know nothing at all about Mrs. Lane (or about Mr. Lane—and because he was on a picnic and dressed casually, you cannot even guess at his socio-economic circumstances).

THE SETTING

Mrs. Lane has been waiting in the relatives' room in the ER for about an hour. The ER has been busy with other cases, so you do not know if she has been seen by any of the staff.

Preinterview Plans

This is the most difficult situation in breaking bad news. All that was known before this interview (as in the three actual cases on which it was based) was that the patient had been on a family outing. It can therefore be assumed that the shock for the relative will be devastating.

In the few seconds that it takes to walk along the corridor to the relatives' room, you can go through a R-O-S-E checklist. You recognize (as anybody would!) that this is going to a very hard interview with high emotion and shock. The objectives are straightforward: to share the bad news with Mrs. Lane and support her by acknowledging her intense emotions with empathic responses. Another objective is practical: you will need her to identify someone who can help her get home later.

In regard to the S for Strategy, clearly the CONES approach is going to be useful, but you will need to find out as much as you can about her understanding of the situation as you start.

Finally, just before you go into the room, take a deep breath and exhale as slowly as you can manage. In doing that, you remind yourself that any physician (not just you!) would find this interview difficult.

Points to Watch For

There are two important techniques to use here. First, to introduce yourself (and shake hands). Next, after the opening, try to work out what the relative was thinking about the situation. In this case, Mrs. Lane had been thinking about a food allergy or a seizure as the cause of his collapse, so when she hears that it was a heart attack, she is devastated.

What Could Have Been Done Differently?

How would you (or do you) start such interviews?

Mrs. Lane wonders why the resuscitation attempt was stopped after less than an hour. Was the explanation of electromechanical dissociation appropriate? Too long? Too short? How would you have handled that question?

Do you think it's a good idea for the relative to view the body?

A.4. "How Long Do I Have?"

The Clinical Situation

Mr. Carr has just started chemotherapy for small-cell lung cancer. There is approximately a 70 percent chance that his tumor will respond, but whether his particular tumor will respond is, of course, not yet known. He wants to know whether he should go ahead and buy a time-share condominium.

Mr. Carr is clearly an intelligent and well-informed man. He worries about things a great deal.

Mr. Carr started chemotherapy only a few days ago. He tolerated it well and has not yet developed alopecia.

Preinterview Planning
You have no idea as to what Mr. Carr wants to talk about today. Hence, you do not especially view this interview as tough. In other words, the ROSE checklist would not have raised a red flag.

Points to Watch For
The patient is pressing the physician to provide prognostic information that is simply not there. In these circumstances, because of the uncertainty, it is important that you do not make the decision for the patient. (As is said in the interview, if the physician makes the decision he will be blamed for all the consequences.) So the important thing is for the patient to reflect on—and express—what kind of a person he is in terms of risk management. In fact, this is the central and the most important topic of the discussion.

What Could Have Been Done Differently?
When the physician says, "Remission lasts for a time," the patient looks away and looks disappointed. Would an empathic response to that reaction have been helpful? How would you have phrased it?

A.5. "But the Surgeon Said He Got It All"

The Clinical Situation
Mrs. Wright (another Mrs. Wright, not the same person as the one in scenario 1!) is a new referral to the medical oncology clinic. She was recently diagnosed with node-positive breast cancer, which is routinely treated with chemotherapy.

THE PATIENT
Mrs. Wright is a pleasant and highly intelligent woman.

THE SETTING
She is coming to see you in one of your regular breast cancer clinics.

Preinterview Planning

Before you start the interview, it does not seem to you that this is going to be a particularly difficult interview. Hence, you will probably be thinking that the SPIKES protocol will be the most suitable way of discussing the diagnosis and the treatment plan.

Points to Watch For

When you ask her for her perception of the situation, it becomes clear that she has the impression that surgery was all she needed. She is not sure why she has been sent to you.

What Could Have Been Done Differently?

What would have happened if you had said, "Well, the surgeon got it wrong. He simply doesn't understand breast cancer properly"? How would the interview with Mrs. Wright have proceeded from that point?

A.6. "My Mother's Not to Be Told"

The Clinical Situation

Mrs. Geffin is a woman in her mid-60s who has been referred to you for recommendations about her newly diagnosed breast cancer (according to the referral note). However, before you have even met her, her son, who is in his early 30s, comes into the consultation room (while his mother is still outside in the waiting area).

THE SON

Mrs. Geffin's son is clearly highly intelligent and articulate and has definite ideas about how the situation with his mother should be handled.

THE SETTING

You weren't expecting this! Mrs. Geffin's son comes into the consultation room when you were expecting his mother.

Points to Watch For

The objective is to help the patient's son come around to a different course of action from the one he arrived with. To do this, his role as his mother's support needs to be emphasized and reinforced.

What Could Have Been Done Differently?

What would have happened if you had stuck to the regulations and simply refused to consider his demands about his mother?

The Clinical Situation

THE PATIENT

Mr. Carter is a 52-year-old man who has small-cell lung cancer. He completed six courses of chemotherapy, and the disease went into complete remission with no detectable evidence of tumor.

Statistically, this happens frequently, as he was told, and approximately 15 percent of patients will still be in remission two years after starting chemotherapy, although unfortunately most of those will succumb to recurrent progressive cancer thereafter.

THE SETTING

Mr. Carter is attending today just about two years after starting chemotherapy. There is no evidence of disease on his most recent CT scan of lungs.

Points to Watch For

Mr. Carter is clearly delighted with his situation and feels that a threshold has been crossed and that he is cured. You know that, sadly, this is highly unlikely and that it is most likely that his disease will recur. You want to support and reinforce his mood without promising or guaranteeing that the remission will last in the long term.

What Could Have Been Done Differently?

Mr. Carter is incorrect when he claims that he has been cured. Would it have been possible to confront his statement directly? If so, what would have happened in the interview following that?

A.8. The Last Interview: Saying Goodbye

The Clinical Situation

Mrs. Anderson was diagnosed with breast cancer four years ago. It has recurred in the bone marrow, causing a leukoerythroblastic anemia a few months ago. After a brief response to Adriamycin, the disease is now progressing, and she has been admitted to the hospital palliative care unit (there being no domestic palliative care services available at that time).

THE PATIENT

Mrs. Anderson has been your patient for several years. She has always faced her clinical situation appropriately and bravely. She has two children in their teens with whom you discussed her situation (at her request and with her present).

She has become very fatigued with the anemia and is now asleep for much of the time.

Points to Watch For

It is permissible and helpful to tell the patient that she has always shown bravery and resourcefulness in the face of progressive disease.

What Could Have Been Done Differently?

Would it have helped to paint a more optimistic picture of the situation? What would have happened over the ensuing days if you had done that?

Notes

··

Chapter One. Some "Can't Go Wrong" Tips

1. Hall, E. T. 1966. *The Hidden Dimension*. Garden City, NY: Anchor.

2. Schertz, J. W., Edwards, H. T., and Kallail, K. J. 1995. *Communicative Effectiveness of Doctor-Patient Interactions, Health Communication*, Vol. 7. San Francisco, CA: Routledge.

3. Beckman, H. B., and Frankel, R. M. 1984. The effect of physician behavior on the collection of data. *Annals of Internal Medicine* 101:692–96.

4. Russell, J. A., and Fernandez-Dol, J. M., eds. 1997. *The Psychology of Facial Expression*. New York: Cambridge University Press.

5. Pollak, K. I., Arnold, R. M., Jeffreys, A. S., Alexander, S. C., Olsen, M. K., Abernethy, A. P., Sugg Skinner, C., Rodriguez, K. L., and Tulsky, J. A. 2007. Oncologist communication about emotion during visits with patients with advanced cancer. *Journal of Clinical Oncology* 25 (36): 5748–52.

6. Morse, D. S., Edwardsen, E. A., and Gordon, H. S. 2008. Missed opportunities for interval empathy in lung cancer communication. *Archives of Internal Medicine* 168 (17): 1853–58.

7. Eva, K. W., Rosenfeld, J., Reiter, H. I., et al. 2004. An admissions OSCE: The multiple mini-interview. *Medical Education* 38:314–26. Mercer, S. W., Maxwell, M., Heaney, D., et al. 2004. The consultation and relational empathy (CARE) measure: Development and preliminary validation and reliability of an empathy-based consultation process measure. *Family Practice* 21 (6): 699–705.

8. Korsch, B., and Negrete, V. 1972. Doctor-patient communication. *Scientific American* 227:66–73.

9. Buckman, R., and Baile, W. 1998. *A Practical Guide to Communication Skills in Clinical Practice* (CD-ROM set) and 2003. *A Practical Guide to Communication Skills in Cancer Care* (CD-ROM set). Toronto: Cinemedic Productions.

Chapter Two. Breaking Bad News

1. Buckman R. 1984. Breaking bad news: Why is it so difficult? *BMJ* 288: 1597–99.
2. Oken, D. 1961. What to tell cancer patients. *JAMA* 175:1120–28.
3. Cousins, N. 1964. *Anatomy of an Illness as Perceived by the Patient: Reflections on Healing and Regeneration.* New York: W.W. Norton & Co.
4. Shadyac, T., director. 1998. *Patch Adams.* Universal Studios.
5. Buckman, R. 1988. *I Don't Know What to Say: How to Help and Support Someone Who Is Dying.* New York: Random House.
6. Evans, C., and McCarthy, M. 1985. Prognostic uncertainty in terminal care: Can the Karnofsky index help? *Lancet* 1 (8439): 1204–6.
7. Cassell, E. 1990. Hope as an Enemy [lecture], Toronto, March.
8. Buckman, R. 1998. Communication in palliative care: A practical guide. In Doyle, D., Hanks, G.W.C., and MacDonald, N., eds., *Oxford Textbook of Palliative Medicine.* Oxford University Press.

Chapter Three. Disclosing Error

1. Kraman, S., and Hamm, G. 1999. Risk management: Extreme honesty may be the best policy. *Annals of Internal Medicine* 131:963–67.
2. Levinson, W., and Gallagher, T. H. 2007. Disclosing medical errors to patients: A status report. *CMAJ* 177:265–67.
3. Priest, L. 1998. *Operating in the Dark: The Accountability Crisis in Canada's Health Care System.* Doubleday Canada.

Chapter Five. Giving Information Effectively

1. Korsch, B., and Negrete, V. 1972. Doctor-patient communication. *Scientific American* 227:66–73.
2. In general terms, the borderline personality is a personality type (and so not curable) in which personal relationships are not maintained, and the person's needs are multiple and in practical terms unrealizable.

Chapter Six. Some Particularly Difficult Conversations

1. Buckman, R. 1998. Communication in palliative care: A practical guide. In Doyle, D., Hanks, G.W.C., and MacDonald, N., eds., *Oxford Textbook of Palliative Medicine.* Oxford University Press.
2. Buckman, R., and Senn, J. 1990. CPR: Is every death a cardiac arrest? *CMAJ* 142 (2): 155–56.

Index

communication strategies (*cont.*)
related to transition to palliative
care, 113–14; related to what patient
has been told by another doctor,
117–18, 133–34; ROSE protocol to
prepare for difficult conversation,
120–25; SAFER protocol for giving
information to patient, 96–105;
sensitive decisiveness, 19; SPIKES
protocol for breaking bad news,
21–73; with terminally ill patients,
66–73; time management and, 4–6,
18, 104–5; usefulness of, 6–7, 8
comprehension of patient, 31, 37–38;
children, 65
compromise, 94
CONERS protocol, 106–13; Context
(step 1), 108; Opening (step 2),
108–9; Narrative (step 3), 109;
Emotions and enquiries (step 4),
109–11; Request (step 5), 111–13;
Strategy (step 6), 113
CONES protocol, 7, 74, 75, 76, 77,
78–87; for disclosing adverse events,
89; for discussing death, 107;
empathic response in, 83–85; to
inform relatives of patient's death,
87–89; to inform relatives of patient's
deterioration, 89; Context (step 1),
79; Opening remark (step 2), 79–81;
Narrative (step 3), 81–83; Emotions
(step 4), 83–85; Strategy and
summary (step 5), 85–87
conflict: de-escalation of, 94; escalation
of, 91–92; HARD strategy for
management of, 7, 90, 91, 92–95;
limbic system activation and, 91;
warning signs of, 92
contextual learning, 100–101, 104
crying, 55–57
cure: displacement behavior and quest
for, 59–60; hope for, 70

de-escalation, 94
denial, 31–32, 46, 47
depression, 57–58
despair, 46, 54–55
disbelief, 41, 48, 54

displacement behavior and "the quest,"
47, 48–49, 58–60
distance between doctor and patient, 10,
12, 30, 80, 99
doctor-patient relationship, 1–3
do not resuscitate (DNR) orders,
114–16
DVD notes, 129–36; disclosing error,
130–31; estimating survival time,
132–33; family who don't want
patient to be informed of diagnosis,
134; informing relative of patient's
death, 131–32; last interview: saying
goodbye, 135–36; recurrence of
bowel cancer, 129–30; unrealistic
hope, 135; what a patient was told
by another doctor, 133–34
dying and death, 71–73; CONERS
protocol for requesting autopsy
or organ donation after, 106–13;
CONES protocol for discussing, 107;
death denial, 26–27; DNR orders,
114–16; end-of-life decisions, 71–73;
estimating survival time, 66–68,
132–33; euphemisms for, 88;
expressing sorrow for, 108; fear of,
47; hope and, 68–70; informing
family of patient's death, 87–89, 109,
131–32; related to medical error,
82–83; transition to palliative care,
72, 113–14

emotions: adaptive, 46; of doctor after
patient's death, 88–89; empathic
response to, 13–15, 25, 40–43, 83–85,
102–4, 110–11; identification of, 13,
40–41, 84, 102–3, 110; identifying
cause of, 13–14, 41, 84, 103, 110;
maladaptive, 46–47; nonjudgmental
response to, 42; as reaction to bad
news, 21, 23–24, 46–66; as reaction
to error disclosure, 83–85; as reaction
to information, 102; related to request
for autopsy or organ donation,
109–11; sympathy, 24, 25, 80. *See
also* patient reactions
empathic response, 13–17, 25; difficulty
with, 15–16; doctors' lack of, 16–17;

palliative care, 72, 113–14, 116

patient reactions, 21, 23–24, 46–61; adaptive vs. maladaptive, 46–47; anger, 41, 51–53; crying, 55–57; denial, 31–32, 46, 47; depression, 57–58; despair, 46, 54–55; disbelief, 41, 48, 54; displacement behavior and "the quest," 47, 48–49, 58–60; to error disclosure, 83–85; fear, 47–48, 50–51; guilt, 46–47; hope, 46, 68–70; humor, 46, 60–61; organizing and planning, 46; shock, 41, 48, 49–50; "why me?" 57

patients: answering questions of, 101–2; assessing perception of, 28, 29–32, 34; breaking bad news to, 21–73; checking understanding of, 37–38; empathic response to, 13–17, 25, 40–43, 83–85, 102–4, 110–11; expectations of the future, 21, 54; explaining clinical strategy to, 44; finding out what matters to, 49; giving information to, 36–40, 96–105; informing relatives of death of, 87–89, 109; informing relatives of deterioration of, 89; invitation to share information with, 32–36; nonverbal communication with, 8–12, 30, 80; questions about test results, 35–36, 43; saying goodbye to, 135–36; terminally ill, 66–73; variables affecting health outcome of, 1–2; who don't want to know diagnosis, 27–28, 63–64

perception of patient, 28, 29–32, 34

"person-doctoring," 3

powerlessness, 52

preparing for difficult conversations, ROSE protocol for, 120–25

problem solving, 81–82, 85–87

professional behavior, 2

professional failure, 24

psychological shock, 41, 48, 49–50

questions by patients: related to what they were told by another doctor, 117–18, 133–34; responding to, 101–2; about survival time, 66–68, 132–33; about test results, 35–36, 43

red flags: for conflict, 92; for difficult conversations, 122

relaxed appearance, 9–10

ROSE protocol, 120–25; Recognize high stakes interviews in advance (step 1), 122–23; Organize objectives (step 2), 123; Strategize (step 3), 123–24; Exhale (step 4), 124

SAFER protocol, 96, 98–105; Setting and starting (step 1), 98–99; Agenda (step 2), 99–100; Facts (step 3), 100–101; Enquiries and emotions (step 4), 101–4; Reinforcers and wrap-up (step 5), 104

saying you are sorry, 25, 79–80, 108

sensitive decisiveness, 19

setting for conversation, 28–29, 98–99

shaking hands, 9, 12, 30, 80, 86, 99

shock, 41, 48, 49–50

silence, 11, 12, 56

smiling, 11–12, 30, 80, 99

SPIKES protocol, 7, 20, 21, 26, 28–46; vs. CONES protocol, 78; for discussions about transition to palliative care, 114; Setting and starting (step 1), 28–29; Perception (step 2), 28, 29–32; Invitation (step 3), 32–36; Knowledge (step 4), 28, 36–40; Emotions (step 5), 40–43; Strategy and summary (step 6), 44–46

stress, somatic signs of, 92

support for patient/family, 61–62

sympathy, 24, 25, 80

system failure analysis, 75–76

technical jargon, 39–40, 100

telephone contact number, 86

terminal illness, 66–73; acknowledging uncertainty of, 67–68; DNR orders and, 114–16; end-of-life decisions and, 71–73; estimating survival time for, 66–68, 132–33; hope and, 68–70; transition to palliative care for, 72, 113–14. See also dying and death

Robert Buckman has also produced a 38-page, spiral-bound, small-format aide-mémoire for difficult conversations in medicine. To order a copy of *Practical Plans for Difficult Conversations in Medicine: The Pocket Guide*, please contact:

Cinemedic Distributors, Inc.
Box 43172
3980 Grand Park Drive
Mississauga, Ontario L5B 4A7
Canada

Web: www.cinemedic.com
Toll free: 1-877-607-8234
Email: cinemedic@bellnet.ca